CONQUERING DAILY HEADACHE

Alan M. Rapoport, MD
Fred D. Sheftell, MD
Stewart J. Tepper, MD
Andrew M. Blumenfeld, MD

2008
DECKER DTC
HAMILTON

Decker DTC
P.O. Box 620, L.C.D. 1
Hamilton, Ontario L8N 3K7
Tel: 905-522-7017; 800-568-7281
Fax: 905-522-7839; 888-311-4987
E-mail: info@bcdecker.com
www.bcdecker.com

© 2008 BC Decker Inc.

All rights reserved. No part of this publication may be reproduced, stored in a retrieval system, or transmitted, in any form or by any means, electronic, mechanical, photocopying, recording, or otherwise, without prior written permission from the publisher.

08 09 10/WPC/9 8 7 6 5 4 3 2 1

ISBN 978-1-896998-32-9
Printed in the United States by Walsworth Publishing Company
Production Editor: Margaret Holmes; Typesetter: Norm Reid; Cover Designer: Design Intervention

Sales and Distribution

United States
BC Decker Inc
P.O. Box 785
Lewiston, NY 14092-0785
Tel: 905-522-7017; 800-568-7281
Fax: 905-522-7839; 888-311-4987
E-mail: info@bcdecker.com
www.bcdecker.com

Canada
McGraw-Hill Ryerson Education
Customer Care
300 Water St.
Whitby, Ontario L1N 9B6
Tel: 1-800-565-5758
Fax: 1-800-463-5885

Foreign Rights
John Scott & Company
International Publishers' Agency
P.O. Box 878
Kimberton, PA 19442
Tel: 610-827-1640
Fax: 610-827-1671
E-mail: jsco@voicenet.com

Japan
United Publishers Services Limited
1-32-5 Higashi-Shinagawa
Shinagawa-Ku, Tokyo 140-0002
Tel: 03 5479 7251
Fax: 03 5479 7307

UK, Europe, Middle East
McGraw-Hill Education
Shoppenhangers Road
Maidenhead
Berkshire, England SL6 2QL
Tel: 44-0-1628-502500
Fax: 44-0-1628-635895
www.mcgraw-hill.co.uk

Singapore, Malaysia, Thailand, Philippines, Indonesia, Vietnam, Pacific Rim, Korea
Elsevier Science Asia
583 Orchard Road
#09/01, Forum
Singapore 238884
Tel: 65-737-3593
Fax: 65-753-2145

Australia, New Zealand
Elsevier Science Australia
Customer Service Department
Locked Bag 16
St. Peters, New South Wales 2044
Australia
Tel: 61 02-9517-8999
Fax: 61 02-9517-2249
E-mail: customerserviceau@elsevier.com
www.elsevier.com.au

Mexico and Central America
ETM SA de CV
Calle de Tula 59
Colonia Condesa
06140 Mexico DF, Mexico
Tel: 52-5-5553-6657
Fax: 52-5-5211-8468
E-mail: editoresdetextosmex@prodigy.net.mx

Brazil
Tecmedd Importadora E Distribuidora
De Livros Ltda.
Avenida Maurílio Biagi, 2850
City Ribeirão, Ribeirão Preto –
SP – Brasil
CEP: 14021-000
Tel: 0800 992236
Fax: (16) 3993-9000
E-mail: tecmedd@tecmedd.com.br

India, Bangladesh, Pakistan, Sri Lanka
CBS Publishers & Distributors
4596/1A-11, Darya Ganj
New Delhi-2, India
Tel: 232-71632
Fax: 232-76712
E-mail: cbspubs@vsnl.com

Notice: The authors and publisher have made every effort to ensure that the patient care recommended herein, including choice of drugs and drug dosages, is in accord with the accepted standard and practice at the time of publication. However, since research and regulation constantly change clinical standards, the reader is urged to check the product information sheet included in the package of each drug, which includes recommended doses, warnings, and contraindications. This is particularly important with new or infrequently used drugs. Any treatment regimen, particularly one involving medication, involves inherent risk that must be weighed on a case-by-case basis against the benefits anticipated. The reader is cautioned that the purpose of this book is to inform and enlighten; the information contained herein is not intended as, and should not be employed as, a substitute for individual diagnosis and treatment.

Dedications

To my entire family, including Arja, my wife of 41 years, my 3 children, TJ, Mark and Sabrina, their spouses, and my four current and all future grandchildren: my thanks to all of you for consistently supporting my long-time efforts to help advance headache medicine around the world. To my patients: my thanks for having entrusted me with your care.

Alan Rapoport

To all my families: my wife Karen, my son Jason, and my daughter Lauren for their support, love, and encouragement through the years, and of course Joe and Wilma who started it all; to my patients, for their courage, persistence, and partnership in their struggle with this potentially disabling headache disorder; and to my colleagues and patient advocates throughout our country and throughout the world for their contributions and dedication in making this world a better place for headache sufferers: my thanks to all of you.

Fred Sheftell

To my wife, Deb, and my sons, Clinton and Sam: your help and love inspire me continually. To my parents, Clifford and Cynthia.

Stew Tepper

To my mother, Taubelle, and my daughters, Cathy and Betsy, who all suffer from migraine. With love to my wife, Jeanne, and my father, Victor, whose support has always allowed me to achieve my goals.

Andrew Blumenfeld

Contents

Preface, v

1. **Why This Book? Epidemiology, Prevalence, and Impact,** 1
2. **Historical Background,** 4
3. **Diagnosis and Classification,** 8
4. **Causes and Risk Factors,** 17
5. **When to Worry about Your Headaches,** 29
6. **Treatment,** 39
7. **A Final Word,** 55

Index, 57

Preface

Until this one, no book that focused on daily headaches had yet been written specifically for patients. Since this a most disabling form of headache due to its constancy and longevity, our patients need to know the latest in research, diagnosis, and effective treatment for this debilitating condition. The three authors of *Conquering Headache*, Doctors Rapoport, Sheftell, and Tepper, have partnered with Dr. Blumenfeld to bring you a concise and up-to-date review of what is known about chronic daily headache.

The World Health Organization (WHO) has shown that episodic migraine is one of the top 20 disabling disorders on our planet. The burden of illness and costs for migraine are greater than that for epilepsy, stroke, Parkinson's disease, multiple sclerosis, and Alzheimer's disease combined! You can imagine, then, what problems the frequent and chronic form of migraine called chronic daily headache can cause for the 4% of our population that suffers from it daily. Although these headaches are not life threatening, because they occur from 15 to 30 days per month there is no respite from them. They cause enormous pain and disability, severely impacting the lives of our patients and all those close to them.

We know that chronic daily headache disrupts your daily routine, prevents you from planning what you need to do, impacts your job and family, and severely impairs your quality of life. Although the majority of individuals with frequent headaches do not have brain tumors, aneurysms (weaknesses in the walls of the blood vessels in the head), bleeding in the brain, allergies, sinus infections, or significant dental problems, recent studies suggest that frequent migraine may be a progressive disorder for some patients, so controlling it **now** is important.

The most common types of headache are migraine (12% of the population), tension headache (more than 90% of the population), and, to a much lesser extent, cluster headache (less than 0.1% of the population). Chronic daily headache usually develops from migraine, and once it is established it is hard to abolish—but it **can** be effectively treated and controlled in most cases.

Although psychological factors play a role in all types of medical disorders, there still is too much emphasis on these issues as the cause of headache. Chronic daily headache is a physiological disorder based in the brain, but it can be influenced by psychological factors such as depression and anxiety.

In this book, you will find the information you need to conquer your chronic headaches and improve the quality of your life. You will learn about many new therapeutic techniques and find up-to-date information about both the epidemiology and the impact of chronic daily headache, the new diagnostic categories, and the process we use to make an accurate diagnosis. You will find reliable information about treating medication overuse headache ("rebound headache") and obtaining optimal acute and preventive treatment. You will be updated about novel devices and procedures such as the occipital nerve stimulator and injections such as botulinum toxin type-A (Botox). You will also discover if you have any of the red flags that would prompt your doctor to suggest further testing to be sure that your headaches do not have a different, organic cause.

The record-keeping system (calendars or diaries) described in this book is similar to the one we give to our patients. It includes our original headache calendar to monitor your headache progress, medication intake and effectiveness, level of disability and headache triggers; and for women, a method to monitor menstrual cycles and hormone replacement therapy.

This book shares state-of-the-art knowledge about headache and dispels many common myths. Here are some basic facts:

1. Headaches are *NOT* all in your head but usually have physiologic causes.
2. Sinus infections and allergies are *NOT* frequent causes of daily headache.
3. Stress is *NOT* a *cause* of headache but rather a contributor to headache.
4. Most daily headache sufferers do *NOT* have temporomandibular joint (TMJ) syndrome as a significant cause.
5. More medication for the acute treatment of headache usually is *NOT* better treatment. In most cases, less medication, taken optimally and early, may offer greater relief.

Finally, this book points the way to the most significant truth about headaches:

6. **You do not have to suffer with headaches. You have to learn to control them so they won't control you!**

This first edition of *Conquering Daily Headache* should not be used to self-diagnose or self-medicate but to inform you about diagnoses and treatment, so that you can better communicate with your doctor and take an active role in your own improvement.

Remember, **you** are in charge and to conquer your daily headaches **you** must take an active role in your own recovery. This book offers information and guidelines to enable you to do exactly that. Good luck!

Alan Rapoport, MD
Fred Sheftell, MD
Stewart Tepper, MD
Andrew Blumenfeld, MD

November 2007

1

Why This Book? Epidemiology, Prevalence, and Impact

"Doctor, my head hurts *all* the time. I wake up with pain and I go to bed with pain. Sometimes it's so bad I feel nauseous and throw up. I have to lie down in a dark room and go to sleep if I can." This vivid description is from a patient with the most common type of chronic daily headache seen in the offices of specialists and headache clinics. It is surely the most challenging and difficult headache type seen by primary care providers.

Chronic migraine or poorly managed chronic daily headache of any type impacts the individual, the family, friends, and the workplace, at high personal and economic cost. Some sufferers struggle through each day to stay functional. Others lead a "bed-to-couch" existence, leaving their homes only to visit various doctors. Frequently they are seeking treatment not only for their headaches but also for the depression and anxiety that accompany chronic daily headache in more than 50% of sufferers.

The spouse of one patient said, "When I tell people my wife had a headache every day of her life, for *years*, they look at me in

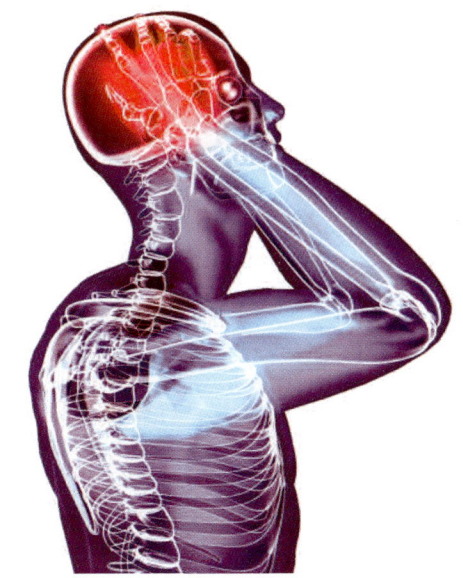

total disbelief!" Yet this is not uncommon. Chronic daily headache, particularly chronic migraine (our focus in this book), occurs on 15 to 30 days per month, and most of the patients seen in headache clinics with this disorder rarely have pain-free days. The majority of patients have a past history of intermittent migraine (hence the term "transformed" migraine, coined by Dr. Ninan Mathew to reflect the "transformation" from intermittent to chronic migraine). A small percentage of patients develop a headache that literally never goes away. The majority of patients who present to headache clinics are overusing a variety of over-the-counter (or more accurately, "off-the-shelf") or prescription medications in an effort to cope.

Headaches are often accompanied by other symptoms that have a major impact on people's lives:

- Difficulty falling asleep or staying asleep
- Fatigue
- Decreased ability to enjoy the things they used to
- Problems with memory and concentration
- Decreased interest in sexual activity.

In addition, sufferers may lose their jobs, family life is disrupted, and they have a decreased overall quality of life. One study showed that the average headache frequency over a 3-month period can approximate 85 days at the high end of the range, with performance affected on over 50 of those days.

A scale that was developed by doctors to assess the impact of chronic headache, the MIDAS (**MI**graine **D**isability **A**ssessment **S**cale) Questionnaire, developed by Prof. Richard Lipton and Dr. Walter Stewart, showed scores of up to 73 in patients with this condition. The cutoff for severe disability on this scale is 20. The scale measures missed or diminished performance related to work or school, ability to perform routine household chores, and social activities. The impact of chronic headache is measured by the overall effect on individuals and their families. If one's ability to function ceases or is markedly diminished, significant others will need to come home and care for small children, and co-workers will need to absorb the workload of the sufferer. Young children may become "parentified," meaning that they will assume parental responsibilities for the parent sufferer and/or younger siblings. One patient recalled taking her 6-year-old daughter to the funeral of her uncle, who was being viewed in an open casket and being buried with his hat and cane (he was a fine Irish gentleman). The daughter tugged at our patient's hand and whispered, "Mommy, when they bury you will you have your ice-pack?"

Migraine-related headache is ranked by the World Health Organization as one of the top twenty disabling disorders on our planet and the eleventh leading cause of disability amongst women. The economic cost reaches billions of dollars, including both direct costs (such as individual medical visits; emergency room visits; medication) and indirect costs (such as diminished or lost productivity at work).

The prevalence of chronic daily headache, although small in the general population (about 4% in most studies, with half of those having chronic or "transformed" migraine), is large in specialty headache clinics. One study in a headache center showed that close to 80% of patients with chronic daily headache actually suffered from chronic or transformed migraine, about 15% from chronic tension-type headache, and 5% from rarer forms of chronic daily headache ("hemicrania continua" or new daily persistent headache). These are described in Chapter 3.

To summarize, chronic daily headache (occurring more than 15 days per month and lasting at least 4 hours) is prevalent in the general population and is the most common headache type seen in the office of headache specialists. Its impact is considerable, not only on sufferers but on their families, friends, and co-workers. Management of chronic daily headache presents a significant challenge. Although treatment may take time and may present difficulties, there is no need to despair. This is *not* a disorder that "you have to learn to live with." We will review the many opportunities for treatment, both pharmacologic and non-pharmacologic, that are currently available.

2

Historical Background

An intriguing article, "Chronic Migraine and Medication-Overuse Headache Through the Ages," appeared a few years ago in the journal *Cephalalgia* (a word that means "head pain"), written by Drs. Chris Boes and David Capobianco. It outlined how Sir Thomas Willis, who coined the term "neurology" and described what is now known as the "circle of Willis" (an important convergence of key blood vessels at the base of the brain) was one of the first to describe chronic daily headache, way back in 1672. Willis was a contemporary of Sir William Harvey, who made important contributions to describing the circulatory system in the body. Sir William had a patient who did not respond to any headache treatment, despite his best efforts (this may sound familiar to present-day readers). He then referred the patient, a countess, to his friend and colleague, Dr. Willis, for trepanation (or "trephination"): this meant drilling holes in her skull to treat her chronic headaches as shown in the picture at right. (Some of our readers might be willing to try that if it guaranteed a cure, but please don't!) Trepanation was one of the first treatments for headache; its aim was to release the evil spirits, a procedure that was abandoned as people learned more about the nature of headache

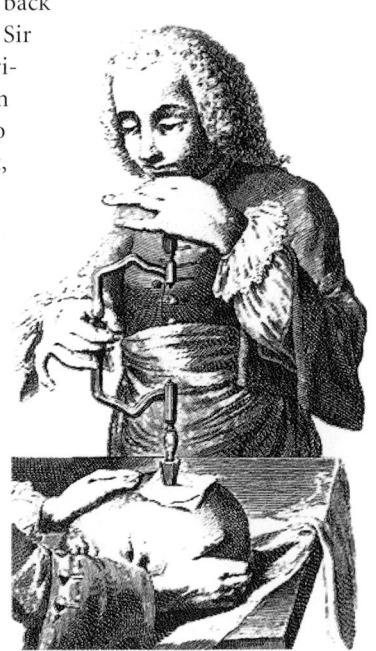

and treatment skills advanced. Dr. Willis thought this approach barbaric and refused to perform the procedure. Sir William then sent the countess to colleagues in France; we learn that she survived the procedure but fared no better. Willis described her headaches as follows: "Formerly, the fits came not but occasionally and seldom under 20 days a month, but afterwards they came more often, and lately she was seldom free….she was cruelly tormented with them." Willis was describing what we now call "transformation" from intermittent to chronic migraine, the most common form of chronic daily headache seen in headache clinics. This accurate description of chronic migraine was offered and observed by Willis almost 350 years ago!

Little information describing chronic daily headache is found until the late 19th and early 20th centuries. Dr. Hermann Oppenheim of Germany described "a form of migraine which is characterized by the *constancy of the head-pain*" and went on to say, "Its chief point of differentiation is that it occurs in persons who have suffered from typical attacks for a long time, or whose parents were troubled with true migraine." Again, this observant doctor noted that many of these patients with chronic daily headache began with intermittent migraine or had a family history of migraine. Interestingly, he also noted "the conversion of migraine attacks, particularly in *neurasthenic or hysteric persons.*" Nowadays we believe that what he observed was not that personality issues caused this conversion to chronic daily headache, but that these disorders may be associated with depressive or anxiety disorders, largely secondary to shared neurologic or brain mechanisms.

In 1922, James Collier commented: "In some cases of longstanding [migraine], the attacks become less severe towards middle life, and a persistent aggravating headache may develop between the attacks. When such a persistent headache is complained of alone, it is very important to inquire about preceding migraine, for the same treatment is applicable to the two conditions." Modern studies have proved Dr. Collier correct in that many people with frequent migraine develop less severe episodes over the years, with a reduction in associated symptoms (vomiting, nausea). The headaches may even resemble tension-type headache (non-throbbing, felt on both sides, without vomiting, mild to moderate pain), and the medications used to treat these headache types are similar or identical to those used to treat migraine. Most researchers in the Americas believe migraine and tension-type headache to have similar origins, while most Europeans see them as separate disorders.

Dr. Ray Baleat, an allergist from the University of Oklahoma, in 1933 offered a description quite similar to the description from the patient in the opening lines of our first chapter: "In a few patients during the late thirties or early forties we have observed a change from the typical hemicrania [half the head] to chronic headaches, less severe and usually generalized in character. As a rule these patients are never quite free from their headaches. However, they have periods of definite increase in severity, which correspond largely to the attacks that they had been accustomed to having…about 5% of all our cases fall in this classification." What

Dr. Baleat describes here is chronic daily background headache with superimposed episodes of full-blown migraine, *exactly as so vividly described by the patient in the opening lines of this book.*

Dr. William Lenox, in an article published in the *New England Journal of Medicine* in 1934, may have been one of the first to add the issue of medication-overuse headache ("rebound headaches," described in detail in Chapter 4 of this book): "Patients whose attacks are terminated when treatment is first instituted may later on fail, at times, to obtain relief, or else the interval between attacks may be shortened." It is now well established that medication overuse may be a contributing or even a *causative* factor in the development of chronic daily headache and that it is characterized by decreased effectiveness of medications that originally worked. Dr. Mary Sullivan in 1936 went on to observe, "…migraine is a protracted condition and we do not know what serious effects the daily use of the drug over long periods of time may have on our patients." How prophetic!

Drs. Gustavus Peters and Bayard Horton of the Mayo Clinic may have been the first to go beyond the observation of acute medication (in their case ergotamine) and recommend a withdrawal program, over 40 years ago. Addressing medication overuse in patients with chronic daily headache is now an accepted standard of care throughout the world and a staple in our treatment of this disorder. It is also one of the most difficult aspects of treatment for sufferers. It was Arnold Friedman (founder of the Montefiore Headache Clinic in 1945) who in 1955 wrote that withdrawal "should be done in a hospital setting or under strict surveillance at home." More modern strategies for accomplishing the transition from overuse to intermittent use are now available, and for more complex cases this may be done in the context of an interdisciplinary team approach.

Dr. Roland Wörz and colleagues noted in the late 1970s that the continuous use of mixed analgesics could lead to the development or worsening of chronic headache. They accurately described the phenomenon of "rebound" headache: "In the vicious circle of chronic pain and analgesic dependence, an important incentive for repeated drug intake is aggravation of the pain several hours or some days after drug cessation. In the long run, however, the discontinuation of analgesics is often accompanied by a substantial decrease of pain intensity or a change from persistent intermittent pain. Therefore, withdrawal of analgesic drug mixtures is effective and appropriate therapy for some patients with chronic pain."

As we approach the modern-day concepts, we owe a great debt to our friend and colleague, Dr. Lee Kudrow, who founded the California Medical Clinic for Headache in Encino, California in the 1970s. Dr. Kudrow observed that a large percentage of his patients with chronic daily headache *were getting worse in spite of escalating use of pain medications!* He was the first in history to do a prospective study, meaning it was not just an observation but a study done moving forward to examine the hypothesis that discontinuation of analgesics was essential to reduce the frequency and constancy of headache. He took this group and divided it in half;

one half was taken off their offending medication and the other half was left on their medication. He then divided each of those groups into half again and gave one-half the prevailing preventive medication (amitriptyline) and the other half no preventive. The group that did best was the one that was taken off the offending analgesics and given amitriptyline, followed by the group that *was simply taken off the offending analgesics*. The two remaining groups who were left on their offending medication both did poorly. Two crucial factors were learned:

- Improvement requires addressing the overuse of analgesics
- Preventive strategies may be rendered less effective, or even ineffective, in the presence of overuse.

This is a topic of debate, as some studies show that certain pharmacologic agents may be effective in helping to reduce medication overuse. Even so, Kudrow's studies have been replicated throughout the world *with the same results*. Saper in 1983 noted that 80% of patients with chronic daily headache overused acute medications, 80% had a history of intermittent migraine, and frequency of medication (not the amount) was the most important determinant of "rebound."

In a study at the New England Center for Headache published in 2004, it was shown that patients in the large group who were successfully withdrawn from their offending medication achieved a 74% decrease in headache frequency, while those who were not able to stop the offending medication achieved only a 17% decrease in frequency.

And so it appears that chronic daily headache was described as long as 350 years ago and that the issue of medication overuse has been observed for nearly a century. It was not until the appearance of the article by Boes and Capobianco, however, that attention was given to this history, and in fact most modern-day articles do not reference these works (largely because they may not be available in routine literature searches). Nevertheless, both sufferers and providers need to acknowledge and be aware of these contributions to the field of chronic daily headache. We owe a strong debt of gratitude to those who came before us!

3

Diagnosis and Classification

The first step in proper care of a patient with headache is to make a correct diagnosis of all the types of headache that the patient experiences. The biggest obstacle in managing chronic daily headache is realizing that the patient often has *multiple types* of headache, then diagnosing each and treating each successfully. Diagnosing the types and causes of headache in a general practice can prove to be a daunting task given the myriad clinical problems that are seen on a daily basis by a physician not specialized in headache. Sometimes, daily headache is of a particular type, with a specific treatment. It takes up to 30 minutes or more to take an accurate headache history, and general physicians often do not have that much time.

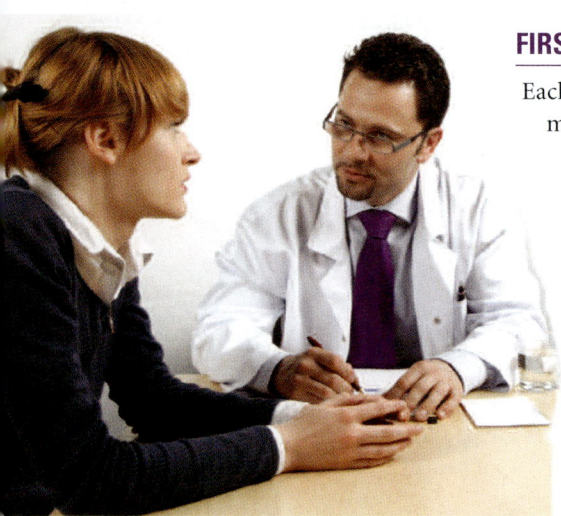

FIRST STEP: TAKING A HISTORY

Each type of the four common primary headaches (migraine, chronic headache, tension-type headache, and cluster headache) is diagnosed from the details that the patient gives the doctor about that headache (Table 3-1). The physician needs to ask many questions about each type of headache that the patient experiences, and delves into each quite deeply. Many doctors start by asking patients an open-ended ques-

Table 3-1: Characteristics of the Four Principal Headache Types

	Migraine	Chronic Daily Headache	Tension-Type Headache	Cluster
Average Starting Age	8–10 YO for boys; 11–14 YO for girls	35–40 YO	20–40 YO	30–40 YO
Frequency	1–3 per month	15 or more days per month	1–30 per month, usually 10/month	1–3× per day when in a cluster period
Location	One eye or temple > both sides	Both sides	Both sides	One eye or temple
Intensity of Pain	Moderate to severe	Mild to moderate, occasionally severe	Mild	Extremely intense, unbearable
Quality of Pain	Throbbing-pounding	Steady > throbbing	Steady, pressing, squeezing	Boring, constant pressure
Associated Symptoms	Occasional tearing and stuffed nostrils both sides	Rare	Rare	Frequent red and tearing eye and running nostril only on the side of the pain
Gender Preference	Females 3× more than males	Slightly more in females	Almost equal	Males 4× more than females

tion like, "Tell me about the types of headaches you have." After the patient has described his or her headaches, the physician asks further questions to obtain accurate information about the following aspects of each one of the headaches the patient experiences:

- What age were you when the headache began?
- How did it progress?
- At what time of the day does it begin?
- Which part of the head is affected?
- Is it a one-sided headache or on both sides?
- What does the pain feel like (for example, dull, steady, throbbing, knife-like)?
- How often does it occur?
- How long does it last?

- How intense is it (mild, moderate, or severe)?
- Are there associated symptoms such as nausea, vomiting, sensitivity to light or sound?
- Is there any worsening with exertion?
- What makes it better or worse?
- How does it affect your life?

Many other facts must be uncovered in the history, such as what medications the patient is on now (both off-the-shelf and prescription medications) and what acute and preventive medications have been tried in the past to treat the headaches. For each medication, the doctor needs to know

- Name
- Strength
- How many pills were taken per day
- For how many days or weeks the pills were taken
- Whether or not the medication helped
- What the side effects were that it caused
- Why it was stopped.

Then the doctor needs to know many details of the past history—medical, surgical, allergic, habit, work, social, psychiatric, and family history. It may be helpful also to know about previous head trauma, seizures, sleep problems, dental problems, jaw pain, depression, specific headache triggers, and whether anyone else in the family has migraine or other headaches.

In addition, in order to diagnose chronic daily headache the doctor needs to know on how many days during the month headaches are present. This requires counting days of not just severe headaches but headache days of any kind or intensity. Furthermore, the doctor will want to determine if this pattern of headaches is recent or whether it transformed from occasional headaches to frequent headaches at a certain time in the past.

SECOND STEP: DOING THE EXAMINATION

The doctor then needs to do a general physical examination, looking at blood pressure and the heart especially, followed by a neurologic examination. This tests for proper functioning of different parts of the nervous system, such as the mental status (for example, memory, orientation, ability to calculate, reason, understand, and speak), the twelve cranial nerves, for example, those controlling vision, hearing, facial expression and eye movements, motor (strength all over the body), sensation (ability to feel pin and touch and cold all over), reflexes, walking and coordination, neck (proper range of movement and presence or absence of pain and tenderness) and status of the blood vessels (especially in the head and neck). The doctor will sometimes also examine the temporomandibular joints (TMJ) and palpate the muscles around the head and neck, assessing for tenderness or thickening of these muscles. The neck position and overall posture are also assessed.

THIRD STEP: MAKING A DIAGNOSIS

On the basis of all the information gleaned, the doctor makes one or a series of headache diagnoses. It might be just migraine without aura or with aura, or it might be several types of headache. If there are more than 15 days a month of headache for at least 3 months, the patient will be diagnosed with some type of chronic daily headache (see "What type of headache do I have?" later in this chapter).

If there are any red flags in the history that are of concern to the doctor (see Chapter 5), then further testing may be needed. This might include some bloodwork to check the white blood cells for infection or the red blood cells for anemia. The doctor or nurse may also look for thyroid problems, diabetes, metabolic problems, Lyme disease, or other medical problems. Tests may be ordered, such as computed tomography (CT or "CAT" scan) looking for bleeding or a tumor, magnetic resonance imaging (MRI scan) to look at the brain in more detail, magnetic resonance angiography (MRA) to look at the arteries in the brain or neck, magnetic resonance venography (MRV) to look at the veins in the brain, or a spinal tap to look for evidence of infection or bleeding or for changes in pressure in the spinal fluid. Sometimes a sleep study will be done to assess for sleep disorders such as sleep apnea.

FOURTH STEP: DISCUSSION BETWEEN PATIENT AND DOCTOR

The doctor then sits with the patient (and others accompanying the patient that day) to discuss the diagnoses and different treatment options. Treatments may consist of acute-care medication, daily preventive medicines, behavioral medicine regimens, injections and procedures, diet, exercise, and over-the-counter vitamins, minerals, supplements, and herbs. Usually, acute treatments will be provided to stop a headache attack, and there may be preventive treatments to reduce the frequency, severity, and duration of attacks. If the preventive treatment is to be in the form of medication, it is to be taken every day. Sometimes, preventive medication can be given just before a vulnerable time for migraine, such as (in the case of menstrual migraine) frovatriptan given daily for just 3 days prior to the anticipated onset of the headache. The patient and doctor should decide together how to proceed. Some patients do not want medications; others want medications only and do not want to do anything on their own, so it is important that these choices be informed and made as a doctor-patient team.

After some discussion about the diagnoses, their causes, and their treatments, the patient may need prescriptions, samples, and further education about how and when to take medications, what *not* to take, how to come off the wrong medications, how to eat, and how to exercise. This can be done by the doctor or by a specially trained nurse, nurse practitioner (NP), or physician assistant (PA). The appropriate tests are then booked and another appointment is made.

In clinical practice, we see that many patients are unable to recall the characteristics and frequency of individual headache attacks. They remember best the most recent or more severe headache attacks. Furthermore, clinical features may change during the course of an attack and from one attack to another, so it is difficult for the patient to be accurate. The use of a headache diary or calendar over time makes it possible for the patient to record the features of each attack and to increase the accuracy of reporting on the frequency and intensity of the attacks. Use of the diary is also vital to help the doctor see how much medication a patient is using, how much disability is associated with the headaches, and what relationship the headaches have to menses in women or to other triggers.

Headache calendars (Figure 3-1) can track frequency, intensity, and clinical features of the attacks. Additional captured data may include concomitant symptoms such as nausea, vomiting, and sensitivity to light and sound as well as responsiveness to acute therapy. The headache calendar is used on a daily basis for a minimum of 30 days until a clear picture can be obtained of the patient's headache diagnoses, characteristics, and patterns of medication use. Specialized headache centers often mail a diagnostic diary to their patients 4 to 8 weeks before the first office appointment. The intent of this type of record-keeping instrument is not to make a diagnosis in the absence of a complete history and examination, but to assist the clinician in the formulation of a working headache diagnosis and treatment plan at the initial visit.

Once the diary has been correctly completed for a sufficient period of time, the patient may be able to switch to a more "user-friendly" headache calendar. Although it is important to collect a great deal of data initially, once the pattern is established we recommend completing headache diaries only once a day, so that the patient does not focus on this throughout the day. At this point, patients should have been educated about the features of their headaches and should be able to enter these specific data into their calendars. Patients are generally instructed to have their calendars readily available and to bring them to their follow-up office visits.

For patients taking preventive medications, the use of a calendar may also help the clinician to gauge the effectiveness of the therapeutic regimen and to discover how often the patient takes acute-care medication such as triptans or pain medicines. Another benefit, demonstrated in clinical trials, is an increased level of satisfaction and a perception of improved communication with the physician in patients who use a headache diary. Patients with frequent headaches are difficult to monitor carefully unless they keep an accurate calendar of their headaches.

CLASSIFICATION: WHAT TYPE OF HEADACHE DO I HAVE?

Most people with occasional severe headaches that last many hours and cause a great deal of disability and trouble functioning have *migraine without aura*. About 20% of

Chapter 3 Diagnosis and Classification   13

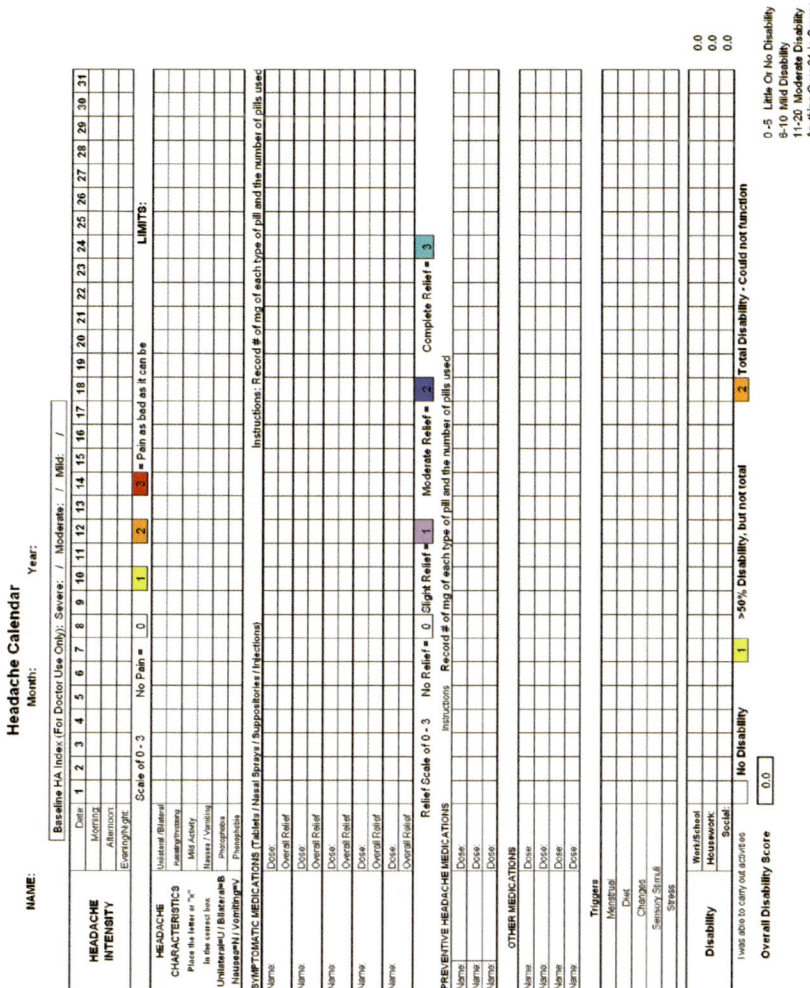

Figure 3-1: Example of headache calendar.

migraineurs have a visual aura prior to their pain that lasts for about 20 to 30 minutes and can take many forms, including colored dots, zigzag lines that blink on and off and move slowly across the visual field, and flashes of light. Migraine is usually an inherited condition, and occurs in 12% of the population, three times more often in women than men. It often presents as a one-sided, severe, throbbing pain associated with nausea and sensitivity to light and sound, causing the patient to need to lie still in a dark, quiet place. This type occurs one to three times per month.

Tension-type Headache

Tension-type headache is much more common, and 40 to 95% of the population has it occasionally. It is a milder headache on both sides, often in the forehead, in or behind the eyes, all over the head, or in the back of the head. It is steady and is not associated with nausea or sensitivity to light or sound. Tension-type headaches are usually trivial and not disabling, and occur from once a month to three times a week.

Cluster Headache

Cluster headache is rare (occurring in 0.1% of the population), and occurs four times more often in men than in women. Occasionally, it is inherited. It causes exquisite pain in and around one eye. Along with the pain, the patient will usually have a red, tearing eye and a stuffed, running nostril on the same side as the pain. The pain usually lasts for 45 to 90 minutes, but comes a few times a day, starting at approximately the same times each day and often waking the patient at night. The pain is excruciating, and is described as a hot poker being thrust into the eye and twirled. It is so severe that patients cannot lie still but rock back and forth or bang the head against a wall. A cluster headache period lasts 4 to 8 weeks and the pain usually disappears for about a year at a time, leaving the patient pain free.

Chronic Daily Headache

Any headache that occurs 15 or more days per month for 3 months or more is called *chronic*, and we have used the term chronic daily headache (CDH). Chronic daily headache is a diverse group of four types of primary headache disorders not related to a structural or systemic illness. These headaches occur 15 or more days per month, last more than 4 hours untreated, and must have been present for more than 3 months. A typical patient with CDH has about 10 days a month with severe headache like a migraine and 20 days per month with a milder tension-type-like headache. Up to 14% of episodic migraine sufferers in one study progressed to develop a chronic form (15 or more days per month) of the disorder. According to the new terminology from the International Headache Society (IHS), subtypes of long-duration CDH now include chronic migraine (CM), chronic tension-type headache (CTTH), hemicrania continua (HC), and new daily persistent headache (NDPH).

Chronic Migraine

Chronic migraine is defined as at least 15 days per month of at least 4 hours per day of pain untreated, with at least 8 days per month at a migraine level or responding to antimigraine medications on those days. Confusingly, international criteria for diagnosing chronic migraine state that this diagnosis can only be made when the patient is not overusing acute medications or caffeine. Chronic migraine is a form of chronic daily headache that is not caused by this overuse, but is rather a transformation from migraine in discrete episodes for reasons that are often not apparent. When a patient transforms to chronic daily headache and is overusing analgesics or caffeine, then the headache is more properly called medication-overuse headache, or analgesic rebound headache, as described in the next section. The results of several analyses indicate that patients with chronic migraine have greater disability and a lower perception of their quality of life than do patients with episodic migraine.

Many patients with CDH are incorrectly diagnosed with migraine only, and the doctor may not realize that this type of headache is complex and difficult to treat.

Medication-Overuse Headache

Risks that increase the likelihood of changing from discrete (separate) episodes of migraine to CDH include a low educational and/or socioeconomic status, obesity, high frequency of headache attacks (more than one day per week), sleep apnea (airway obstruction during sleep), snoring, stressful life events, high caffeine consumption, and, notably, *the overuse of medications designed to get rid of an existing headache*. These medications are also known as "symptomatic," "abortive," or "acute-care" medications. While all of these factors may be important, experts believe that limiting a patient's exposure to acute-care medication may be one of the most effective ways to prevent the progression to CDH.

Many medications that people take for immediate (or acute) relief of migraine headaches can actually make headaches worse if taken too frequently. When this occurs, the resulting problem is called medication-overuse headache (MOH). This was formerly known as "analgesic rebound headache." Generally, experts advise patients to avoid taking acute-care medications (simple or combination analgesics with caffeine, nonsteroidal anti-inflammatory medications, opiates, ergots, or triptans) more than 2 days per week or 10 days per month. We do not know how long it takes to develop this condition, but some suggest it can occur within just a few months.

In the new international headache classification termed ICHD-2, MOH has been most recently defined as headache present on at least 15 days per month, with regular medication overuse (at least 10 days per month) of one or more drugs used for acute and/or symptomatic headache treatment for more than 3 months. In addition, the underlying headache has either developed or markedly worsened during the period of medication overuse. If the headache persists 2 months after withdrawal from overused medications, then a new diagnosis of chronic migraine is given, and the problem was probably not related to the overuse of medication.

New Daily Persistent Headache (NDPH)

This type has no transformation from occasional to frequent headache over months or years, and these patients develop near-daily headaches abruptly. Patients can often remember the exact time that their headaches began and what they were doing. This acute onset of headache may be related to medical tests (myelogram), illness (flu-like conditions) or surgical procedures. This type of headache often has minimal migraine-related features; its features are more similar to those of tension-type headache, but it occurs daily.

In contrast, chronic tension-type headache involves a transformation from occasional to frequent tension-type headache days over months or years.

Hemicrania Continua

Hemicrania continua (HC) is important to recognize, as this type of headache is treatable with an anti-inflammatory medication, indomethacin. This is a headache that is felt strictly over one side of the head and is usually constant and of low to medium intensity. Patients with HC can have some exacerbations or periods of worsening, when the headache becomes more intense for minutes or hours. These exacerbations are usually associated with a droopy eyelid, runny nose, or red and tearing eye on the side of the headache.

CONCLUSION

Most headaches can be diagnosed by means of a careful headache history including other medical conditions as well as the type and number of medicines that the patient is taking. Thorough physical and neurologic examinations can help to rule out more serious causes of headache. Some patients will need further specialized testing. On the first visit the physician should discuss diagnoses and treatment options with the patient, and explain possible side effects of the medications prescribed.

The diagnosis and classification of headache disorders continues to evolve as our understanding of the natural history of chronic daily headache improves. At present, we diagnose CDH in our patients who have headaches at least 15 days per month for at least 3 months. Another common diagnosis in patients with frequent headache is medication overuse headache, which used to be called analgesic rebound headache. This diagnosis is made in patients who are taking acute-care medications at least 10 days per month and whose headaches are worsening or changing because of it. The first part of the treatment in this condition is to slowly stop the overused medication (see Chapter 6).

Although chronic daily headache is complex and at times difficult to diagnose, there is hope for the patient who has been suffering for months or perhaps even years.

Causes and Risk Factors

Our patients frequently ask us, "What causes my headaches?" Another frequently asked question is, "If all my tests are normal and nothing's seriously wrong, why do I get headaches?" Understandably, patients with unexplained symptoms fear the worst, and when most causes of headache have been ruled out, they may fall back on media-driven explanations that attribute headache to sinus, allergy, and stress-related problems. It is not surprising that when test results are normal, many patients fear that their daily headaches are not real but, rather, the result of a psychological process. This is not usually the case.

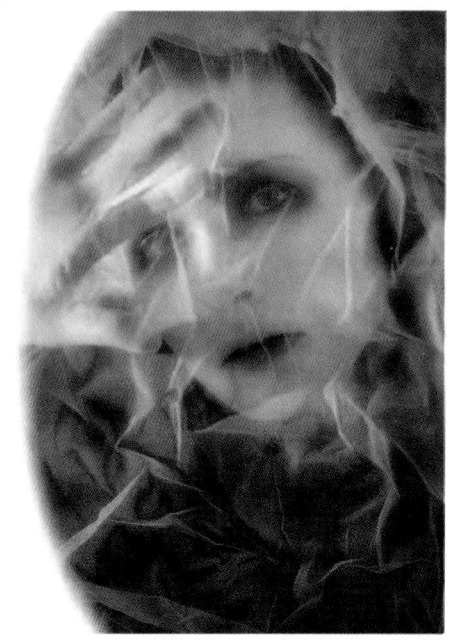

Unfortunately, there are no biologic markers or accurate tests to confirm the diagnosis of the most common headache disorders. Diagnosis of headache is based on a detailed medical history, on neurologic and physical examinations, and on appropriate tests. Most causes of headache probably do not show up on routine tests because we do not yet have the specific means to measure biochemical and electrical changes in the brain, blood vessels, and muscles. Special testing is not always necessary; often headache can be diagnosed by an accurate history and neurologic examination.

HOW TO THINK ABOUT DAILY HEADACHE AND ITS CAUSES

Most daily headaches occur in people who previously had headaches in discrete (separate) episodes. Most of the headaches that precede chronic daily headache are migraine. People notice that their headaches are increasing in frequency, but in adults the experience of transformation is often one of "filling in" the days of no headache with milder headaches. The migraines still occur, but against a background of daily or near-daily lower level headaches. This transformation is rather like raisin bread, where the migraines are the raisins and the background low-level headaches are the bread. The goal of treatment of daily headache is to dissolve away the bread and leave just the raisins, resulting in a patient with migraine in discrete episodes again, and no background headaches. Since most chronic daily headache develops from migraine, some understanding of the causes of migraine is necessary for understanding the causes of chronic daily headache.

CAUSES OF MIGRAINE

Genetics

The tendency to develop migraine is inherited; up to 90% of people with migraine have a close relative who gets them too. Your family history can give your doctor important information that may suggest migraine as a diagnosis. Some studies show that if one parent has migraine, each child has at least a 40% chance of developing it; if both parents have migraine, each child has at least a 75% chance.

The Brain

Migraine begins in the brain, but the pain primarily results from inflammation and from the expansion of blood vessels in the coverings over the brain or meninges. Different experts in headache have different theories on the causes of migraine. These ideas are not mutually exclusive. One widely accepted belief is that the "migraine-prone brain" is too easily excited. According to this theory of a "sensitive" or "hyperexcitable" brain, nerve cells in the brain fire too easily and thereby start the migraine attack. A variety of internal and external trigger factors cause the brain to intitiate a migraine; some triggers are readily apparent (such as fatigue, lack of sleep, too much sleep, stress, weather, and menses), whereas other factors are never found. But the critical understanding is that *it is not the triggers that cause the migraine but rather it is the irritable nerve cells in the brain.*

Low magnesium levels in the brain may be a cause of the abnormal brain electrical activity of migraine. Low magnesium increases the irritability of the nerves, producing electrical changes.

An area of the brain that may be hyperexcitable is the lowest part, called the *brainstem* (Figure 4-1). Nerve cells in the brainstem contain a large amount of a chemical called *serotonin*, which regulates pain. This area of the brain may have a switch or generator that turns on at the beginning of a migraine attack and may cause the migraine to persist for days if not properly treated. The fact that several medications effective in migraine affect serotonin receptors suggests that serotonin may play a crucial role.

Some headache scientists believe that all migraine begins in the cortex, the "thinking" part of the brain. The activation of this area in migraine is called "cortical spreading depression," a term that is not completely accurate because activation comes first, *then* depression! Cortical spreading depression (CSD) is definitely the cause of typical aura, which is a reversible neurologic event lasting more than 5 minutes and less than an hour, and usually followed within an hour by the migraine headache. Aura is often

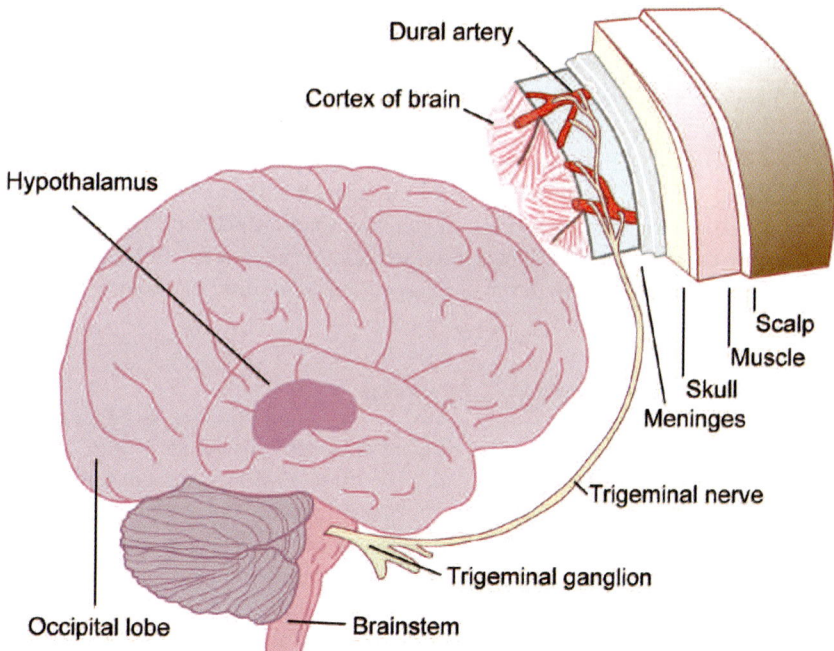

Figure 4-1: Anatomy of brain and scalp showing the trigeminovascular system.

visual, in the form of zigzags, flashing lights, or shimmering blind spots, but occurs in only about one-fifth of migraine sufferers. Whether CSD happens in migraine without aura is controversial. CSD in the cortex may be a generator for all migraine, but this is unresolved.

The Trigeminovascular System

The trigeminovascular system of the brain involves one of the 12 cranial nerves—the trigeminal (or fifth cranial) nerve—and its connections between the arteries in the coverings of the brain (the meninges) and the nerve cells in the brainstem. Research by Dr. Michael Moskowitz showed that chemicals released from the ends of the trigeminal nerve at the meninges cause inflammation to occur around blood vessels, and cause those blood vessels to enlarge and dilate. Many medicines effective in treating migraine—including the triptans and ergots—act at the interface of the trigeminal nerve endings and the vascular system in the meninges by reducing the release of these irritating and dilating chemicals, thereby decreasing the pain.

It may be useful to think of migraine as a process starting in a "central generator" in the upper brainstem that is set incorrectly so that it fires too easily. When this switch turns on, nerves fire and activate the trigeminovascular system, causing inflammation and blood vessel dilation to occur in the meninges. From there, the pain signal goes back into the brainstem, where it is integrated and where nausea and other migraine symptoms are generated.

Therefore, migraine occurs as a three-step process:

1. Activation of the migraine central generator, possibly in the brainstem
2. Activation of the peripheral pain mechanism at the end of the trigeminal nerve in the meninges, resulting in inflammation and blood vessel dilation
3. Re-entry of the pain signals into the brain for integration and initiation of nausea and other migraine symptoms, which last until the "central generator" switch turns off.

CAUSES OF CHRONIC DAILY HEADACHE

People with migraine occurring in discrete episodes can *transform* into having headaches more often than not, that is, more than 15 days per month, which is defined (as noted in Chapter 3) as chronic daily headache. One way to think about chronic daily headache in contrast to migraine, which usually has discrete episodes, is that chronic daily headache transformed from episodic migraine represents the central generator stuck in an "on" position. That is, the generator is activated all of the time, causing headache all or most of the time. The generator may also have a volume control, which goes up and down, accounting for the waxing and waning of headache severity.

Research at Harvard Medical School by Dr. Rami Burstein found a windup or buildup in the brain (called *central sensitization*) of nerve activity during prolonged migraine. This suggests that the sooner a given migraine attack is stopped by medication, the less severe that attack will be. He has also pointed out that many patients whose migraine attacks are not stopped early develop an increased sensitivity of their skin, and actual pain, in response to normal touch, called *cutaneous allodynia*. They describe being unable to comb or brush their hair, to wear a hat, glasses, earrings, or tight collars, or to have anyone touch their skin far into a migraine attack because it hurts them. This correlates with the firing of many nerves in the brain (the central sensitization), and also often also correlates with the triptans not working as well to stop a migraine attack.

It turns out that there is a link between how often someone with migraine has headache days, and the risk of transformation into chronic daily headache. The more days of headache per month, the greater the likelihood of changing from episodic migraine in discrete episodes to frequent headache. When a person with migraine needs to treat 10 or more days of headache per month, that person moves into a critical zone of risk for transformation into chronic daily headache.

It is possible that as the headaches increase, the buildup in the brainstem—the central sensitization—keeps the system going and gradually changes the connections in the brain. This means that the generator is chronically activated in the long term, resulting in chronic daily headache.

The neck and peripheral muscles, even in the scalp and face, offer another entry zone into this system. Dr. Burstein's research demonstrated nerves that connect from the scalp through the skull to the meninges. When the headaches start to occur daily, many patients complain of constant neck and facial pain in addition to the daily headache. Perhaps some of this pain is the allodynia previously mentioned, and debate swirls as to whether the neck and peripheral muscles are triggering headache or are sore due to the headache itself.

One of the chemicals released in the meninges that causes both inflammation and blood vessel dilation is called calcitonin gene-related peptide, or CGRP. This substance is also contained in areas of the brain associated with the trigeminal nerve and pain. Further, CGRP is also released by peripheral nerves of skin or muscle, and may contribute to inflammation in the face, scalp, and neck. It is present in all of the areas involved in the brain, head, and neck that could be involved in the causes of migraine and daily headache.

The approaches to stopping chronic daily headache need to be targeted at all of the potential causes. Daily preventive medications could turn off the central generator. Migraine-specific treatments such as triptans block the release of CGRP and can prevent the inflammation and blood vessel dilation when taken early. Thus, the best timing for use of triptans is *early* in attacks of migraine. This timing can stop attacks completely by preventing the inflammation and blood vessel dilation of the meninges, and by constricting or narrowing the dilated blood vessels. These actions can turn off a migraine completely. However, in the setting of daily headache the usefulness of this approach is limited, because the generator is on continuously.

NEW DAILY PERSISTENT HEADACHE

Sometimes, daily headache can begin without warning and without transformation, that is, on one day, in one place. Patients frequently can remember the exact date of the start of daily headache all at once, and this is referred to as "new daily persistent headache" or NDPH. Presumably, something turns on the generator acutely. When NDPH was first described, it was thought to be related to a viral illness and was called post-viremic headache. However, only about one-third of people with the abrupt onset of daily headache remember a preceding infection or event. For the rest, the cause of the onset of NDPH remains a mystery.

OTHER APPROACHES TO TURNING OFF DAILY HEADACHE

Behavioral techniques may reduce stress and may prevent the activation of the central generator, and can be very helpful in lessening daily headaches. Patients can be taught to use biofeedback and to practice relaxation and stress-reduction techniques, as well as other behavior modification modalities. They can also be taught to regularize lifestyles and to take more time for themselves to decrease headaches.

Injections of botulinum neurotoxin type A (Botox, described in detail in Chapter 6), trigger-point injections, and other injections such as greater occipital nerve blocks can reduce or stop daily headaches, possibly by interrupting the back-and-forth communication between the brain, meninges, and scalp, neck, and muscles. In particular, botulinum neurotoxin type A can reduce CGRP release in the peripheral nerves of the head and neck. This may be another way that botulinum neurotoxin type A can decrease daily headaches.

TRIGGERS

As noted above, triggers do not cause migraine but, rather, turn on the central switch to initiate the process. Many migraine patients are unusually sensitive to internal (within the body) and external (outside the body) changes (Table 4-1). A variety of factors can trigger an explosive migraine attack (Figure 4-2). The menstrual cycle is clearly a significant trigger in the great majority of women with migraine, and this is associated with and may be caused by a decrease in estrogen levels; however, hormonal triggers are rarely a cause of chronic daily headache. A second trigger for migraine is food; many food types can trigger migraine in susceptible patients. While many alcoholic beverages are common triggers, red wine, beer, and champagne are the drinks most frequently mentioned by patients. The dark-colored alcohols (scotch, bourbon, dark rum, and red wine) appear more like-

Table 4-1: Triggers of Migraine

Internal

Chronic fatigue, too little sleep, too much sleep
Change in sleep-wake cycle from travel or shift work
Emotional stress, letdown after the stress is over
Hormonal fluctuations (menstrual cycle)

External

Weather and seasonal change
Travel through time zones
Altitude
Skipping or delaying meals
Sensory stimuli
Flickering or bright lights, sunlight
Odors, including perfume, chemicals, cigarette smoke
Heat, loud noises

Medications

Nitroglycerin
Tetracycline (an antibiotic)
High doses of vitamin A
Some antidepressant medications (selective serotonin reuptake inhibitors or SSRIs)
Some blood pressure medications
Monosodium glutamate (MSG) (a food ingredient)*
Nutrasweet (a food ingredient),** Equal (a sugar substitute),** possibly Splenda (an artificial sweetener) #

*MSG is added to a wide variety of preserved and frozen foods and can trigger migraine. **Food labels should always be carefully read.** Look not only for *MSG* but also for the words *hydrolyzed fat* or *hydrolyzed protein*.

**Both contain aspartame and have been associated with headache in susceptible individuals, especially if taken in large amounts (several diet sodas or other aspartame-containing foods per day).

#Contains sucralose, reported by some headache specialists to trigger migraine.

ly to trigger migraine attacks than the light-colored ones (gin, vodka, white rum, and white wine). Many foods (Table 4-2), particularly those that contain tyramine (such as strong cheddar cheese), trigger migraine, but only in some people. Patients seem to have individual sets of triggers that are problematic for them and not necessarily for others. To reiterate, food triggers bring on migraines, but are not generally a cause of daily headaches.

Caffeine is a double-edged sword. Because caffeine may help constrict the dilated blood vessels during a migraine attack, it is used in combination medicines to increase relief from headache (eg, Excedrin Migraine is a combination of acetylsalicylic acid [Aspirin], acetaminophen [the analgesic in Tylenol], and caffeine; Fiorinal contains caffeine; Cafergot contains caffeine, as does Anacin).

24 CONQUERING DAILY HEADACHE

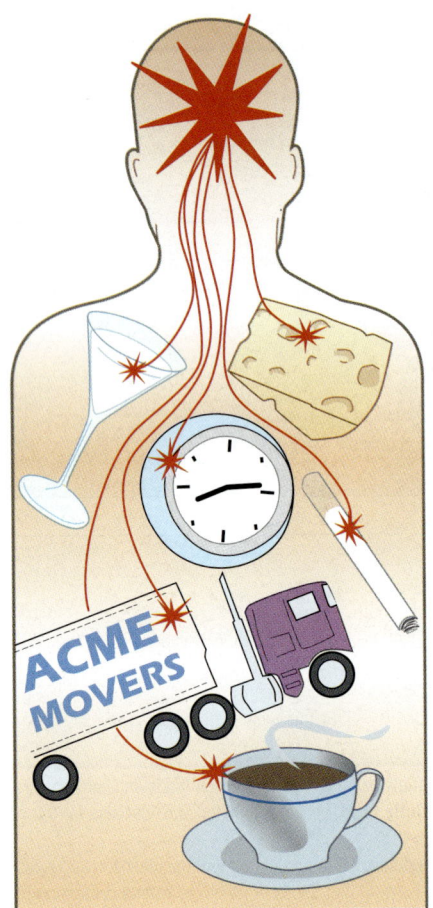

Figure 4-2: Triggers that set off the explosion of migraine.

Table 4-2: Dietary Triggers

Chocolate, onions, Nutrasweet, Equal (aspartame), Splenda (sucralose)
Nuts, pizza, canned figs, peanut butter, avocado, aged cheese
Bananas, processed meats, caffeine (see also Table 4-3)
Alcoholic beverages, eg, red wine
Hot dogs, pepperoni, sausages, bacon, ham, bologna, salami
Pickled or fermented foods
Yogurt
Sour cream

However, habitual consumption of too much caffeine can make headaches worse. How much caffeine is too much? Some patients are sensitive to the small amount of caffeine (approximately 100 mg) in one small (8 oz) cup of strongly brewed coffee. Many patients who complain of headaches on Saturday or Sunday mornings take in less caffeine on weekends than during the week, or sleep later and therefore drink their coffee later in the morning. Headaches that occur under these circumstances could be due to caffeine withdrawal and are more likely to occur in people who are accustomed to drinking more than 300 mg of caffeine per day (about three cups of coffee). At 500 mg per day or above, caffeinism, with symptoms that include disturbed sleep, anxiety, nervousness, rapid or irregular heartbeat, and irritability, may occur. Table 4-3 lists the caffeine content of various products and foods. Gourmet coffees can have over 500 mg of caffeine per large-sized beverage.

Table 4-3: Caffeine Content of Common Foods and Drugs (in mg)

Chocolate, Coffee, and Tea

Chocolate candy bar 25
Cocoa beverage (175 mL mixture) 10
Coffee
   Decaffeinated (150 mL) 2
   Drip (150 mL) 146 (This would be one to two 8 oz cups)
   Instant, regular (150 mL) 53 (This would be about one 8 oz cup)
   Percolated (150 mL) 110 (This is about one 8 oz cup)
   Starbucks regular grande 550
Tea 3-Minute brew (150 mL) 22–46 (This is about one 8 oz cup)

Off-the-Shelf Drugs

Anacin 32
Extra-Strength Excedrin 65
Excedrin Migraine 65 (2 tablets contain 130 mg)
No-Doz tablets 200
Vanquish 33
Vivarin tablets 200

Prescription Drugs

Darvon Compound 65, 32
Esgic 40
Fioricet 40
Fiorinal 40

Soft Drinks (350 mL)

7-Up/Diet 7-Up 0
Coca-Cola 34 (One can)
Diet Coke 45 (One can)
Dr. Pepper 41 (One can)
Mountain Dew 55 (One can)

As noted above, most triggers do not cause daily headache. They can precipitate episodes of migraine, but they are not really causes of migraine either, since the true causes of migraine are the changes in the brain that bring on the attacks.

However, some triggers, such as caffeine (as referred to above), when exposure is frequent, can actually lead to the transformation from occasional headaches to chronic daily headache. That is, if people with migraine consume excessive caffeine frequently or analgesics often, especially those containing caffeine such as Excedrin and Anacin, then these substances actually result in daily headaches. It takes only about 10 days of overuse of these substances per month over several months to make a patient susceptible to this transformation to daily headache. When consumption of these medications is at 10 or more days per month, and the headaches worsen in terms of frequency, severity, or duration, then medication-overuse headache, as a manifestation of daily headache, is likely. Thus, it is important to remember that caffeine is a medication and that overuse of caffeine can lead to a daily headache that is a form of medication-overuse headache—a *caffeine-overuse headache*. Perhaps overuse of caffeine turns on the central generator as a cause of daily headache, or the patient with excessive caffeine use is in constant caffeine withdrawal, thus developing daily headache as a manifestation of daily withdrawal.

STRESS, DEPRESSION, AND ANXIETY

Although stress is high on the list of migraine triggers, it does not usually cause migraine headaches in those who are not biologically predisposed to migraine. Migraine can also occur during letdown periods, such as after the stress has come and gone, or during a period of unwinding or relaxing. This may explain why many patients have migraine attacks on weekends or on vacations.

Another question frequently asked is whether stress can cause daily headaches. Stressful life events in the previous year are associated with a transformation to daily headache. A stressful time in life can increase the frequency of all headaches, and as the number of headache days increases, the risk for daily headaches increases. No one knows why stress increases the likelihood of daily headache, but as discussed above, stress-reducing techniques, such as biofeedback, can help in the treatment of daily headache, speeding the return to headaches in discrete episodes occurring less than 15 days per month.

Depression and anxiety are often associated with chronic daily headache, tension-type headache, and migraine, and should be addressed as part of a patient's entire headache picture. Some patients with depression and anxiety need behavioral treatment from a psychologist, some may need medication, and some may need both. The likelihood of depression or anxiety is also much higher in chronic daily headache, and although chronic daily headache is not considered a psychological illness, treating these accompanying disorders can expedite help for those with chronic daily headache.

OTHER RISKS FOR DEVELOPING CHRONIC DAILY HEADACHE

As noted above, stressful life events, and overuse of medications such as caffeine and analgesics have been related to the onset of chronic daily headache. Dr. Marcelo Bigal showed that obesity and thyroid disease can be associated with the onset of daily headache, and also (as previously stated) infections such as viruses and Lyme disease can trigger daily headache. A search for thyroid abnormalities, infection, and a discussion on the frequency of medication intake with your doctor or care provider is clearly indicated in the setting of daily headache.

Dr. Anne Scher completed a large study that explored and ranked risks for developing daily headache. Some of these are included in Table 4-4, below.

The Neck

Early theories of causes of tension-type headache attributed the pain to contraction of muscles around the head and neck, which explains why this type of headache was originally termed *muscle-contraction headache*. It is true that tension-type headache may occur in people who, for one reason or another, unconsciously tighten up the muscles around the head, neck, and shoulders. All of the following may also be triggers of tension-type headaches or contribute to headaches in general: poor posture, tense jaw, temporomandibular joint problems, arthritis, disk disease in the neck, and occupational factors, such as sitting for long periods at computer terminals, typing, or cradling the telephone between the ear and the shoulder.

Patients with chronic headaches can develop a head-forward posture. This involves forward displacement of the head relative to the shoulders. It usually develops from prolonged deskwork with decreased strength of the back muscles. This can lead to muscle trigger points and referred pain to the head. It is easy to understand how tight muscles could be related to tension-type headache, but factors within the brain may be involved as well, particularly in patients who develop chronic tension-type headache as a form of chronic daily headache. A similar sen-

Table 4-4: Risks for Developing Daily Headache

Medication overuse of at least 10 days per month
High caffeine use
Abnormal thyroid function
Infections, such as viruses and Lyme disease
Headache attack frequency (the more attacks, the more likely the development of daily headache)
Stressful life event(s) in the preceding year
Head injury
Snoring
Obesity
Pre-existing migraine

sitization process to migraine may occur, that is, the gradual transformation from discrete headaches to daily headaches associated with tight or abnormal neck musculature. There remains somewhat of a question as to which comes first, the chicken or the egg—the neck tightness or the headaches. It is nonetheless clear that reduction of neck muscle tension via non-drug therapies, and resolution of neck pain helps with control of all headaches and with resolving chronic daily headache. However, daily headache and tension-type headache may have nothing to do with muscles or tension in some patients.

Possible Connections Between Tension-Type Headache and Migraine

Because some of the symptoms of tension-type headache and migraine overlap, and because many people suffer from both types of headache, several headache specialists believe that these two conditions are related. Many patients may develop an acute tension-type headache that, over a period of hours, evolves into a clear-cut migraine. It is not surprising that one group of headache specialists believes that headaches represent a continuum that includes tension-type headache and migraine, which share similar underlying mechanisms. Another group considers the two headache types to be completely distinct disorders. A third theory is that tension-type headache that occurs in migraine sufferers is really low-level migraine, whereas tension-type headache in people who do not get migraine is a distinct and separate type of headache. One major study supports this third hypothesis.

The link between tension-type headaches and migraine is made even stronger when one thinks about chronic daily headache, since patients can develop chronic daily headache from tension-type headaches or from migraine. In other words, chronic daily headache can begin with episodes of either type and then transform to daily headache.

SUMMARY

Chronic daily headache usually transforms from episodic migraine, often due to overuse of pain medication (analgesics), as-needed medications, or caffeine. The "central generator" for migraine gradually turns on all of the time in most chronic daily headache. An exception is new daily persistent headache, which begins abruptly. All chronic daily headache merits discussion with a care provider to explore causes and solutions.

5

When to Worry about Your Headaches

More than 95% of headaches are primary headaches that are not caused by serious underlying medical conditions. You should, however, be aware of the "red flags" or danger signals listed below, since these are signs that you should seek medical attention.

Doctors use the term "secondary headache" if the headache is due to a medical condition such as infection, tumor, or other problem. The term "primary headache" means that the headache is not due to one of these conditions. Since most headaches are primary, doctors and patients alike must be vigilant for clues to the presence of something potentially life-threatening as a cause of either headaches that occur in episodes or of daily headaches.

Consult a doctor if you experience any of the following:

- You rarely get headaches and suddenly develop a severe one.
- You often get headaches and develop a new type or one that comes on suddenly and remains severe.
- You develop the worst headache you have ever had.
- You are over 40 years old and start to develop headache for the first time.
- You develop a daily headache that gradually worsens over a period of days or weeks.

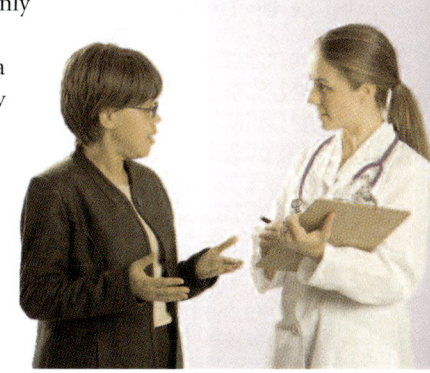

- You get headaches when you exercise, cough, sneeze, strain while having a bowel movement or during other strenuous activities, have sex, or bend over. (They could be exertional migraine or benign exertional headaches, but you may have something more serious.)
- You get a "bug" or virus, and you develop a severe headache accompanied by nausea, vomiting, and such severe stiffness of the neck that you cannot put your chin on your chest without pain. You must seek medical attention right away to rule out meningitis or hemorrhage.
- You get a headache accompanied by any of the following neurologic symptoms: trouble with coordination, double vision, weakness or numbness in any extremity or on one side of the body, drowsiness, inability to stay awake, confusion, impaired speech, or a change in personality.
- You have a serious underlying disease already, including cancer, autoimmune disease such as lupus, or a chronic infection such as human immunodeficiency virus (HIV). With significant underlying illness, headache can be a symptom of a life-threatening problem.
- You have a change in the pattern of your headaches, in terms of frequency, severity, or duration. This includes the *new* onset of daily headache.

DANGER SIGNALS

In general, these should be medically evaluated as soon as possible:

- A new-onset headache in someone who does not usually get headaches
- A headache that is much more severe than usual
- A significant change in a typical headache
- A headache that escalates in severity more rapidly than usual or steadily over many days.

ROLE OF THE HEALTH-CARE PROVIDER

When you visit your own physician or a neurologist or headache specialist, you should be questioned carefully about your headaches. The doctor should ask about each type of headache you have and request details, as listed in Table 5-1.

Keeping a headache diary will allow you to accurately answer these questions. Your doctor will then do a physical and neurologic examination and evaluate your mental alertness, cranial nerve function (including vision, hearing, strength and sensation of the face), strength, coordination, and walking, reflexes, and ability to perceive different sensations. In addition, your blood pressure, pulse, neck range of motion, and the state of the arteries in your head and neck will be evaluated (Figure 5-1).

Table 5-1: Questions that Should Be Asked by Your Health Care Provider

When did the headache/s start?
How frequently do you get this type of headache?
On how many days of the month do you have a headache of any kind?
How long does it last?
How does it impact on your life?
Where is the pain located?
How severe is it?
Are there other symptoms associated with it, such as nausea, vomiting, and sensitivity to light and sound?
Does exertion or even movement worsen the headache?
What brings it on (triggers it)?
What makes it better?
What is your behavior like during the headache?
Has there been a change in your headaches recently?

Although the histories of migraine sufferers and those with daily headache can be dramatic, most people usually turn out to have basically normal neurologic examination results. In fact, people with migraine and chronic daily headache *should* have normal examination results. If there is anything abnormal on examination, the doctor will become concerned that another process may be causing the headaches, that is, that they are in fact, or could be, secondary headaches.

Even if your examination is normal, your doctor may order blood tests to check for infection and inflammation, metabolic problems, liver or thyroid dysfunction,

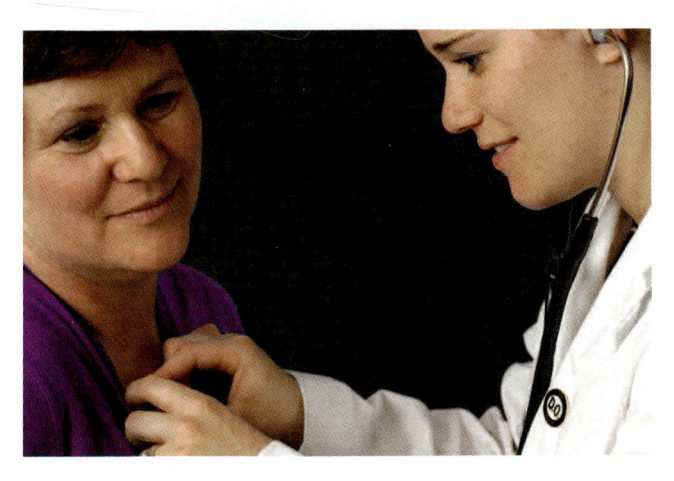

Figure 5-1: The neurologic examination should include listening for abnormal sounds (bruits) in the neck.

Lyme disease (depending on where you live), and other conditions that might contribute to your headaches. Do not be surprised if your doctor sends you for a computed tomography (CT or CAT) scan (Figure 5-2), magnetic resonance imaging (MRI) of your head, or even magnetic resonance angiography (MRA), because these are the best ways to rule out serious structural problems in the brain. CT, MRI, and MRA are painless. CT involves the use of x-rays; an iodine-containing dye may be injected into an arm vein to increase the contrast of the images. Be sure to tell your doctor if you are allergic to iodine.

MRIs and MRAs do not use x-rays; rather, they are done in a strong magnetic field. Another type of dye may be injected into an arm vein. Most MRI machines resemble a small tunnel, open at both ends.

MRIs provide more detailed information about certain areas of the brain. Pregnant women should not undergo either type of scan, but MRI is preferable to CT when imaging is necessary. Be sure to tell your doctor if you are going for an MRI and you have any metal hardware that was placed in your body during previous surgery. For patients who are claustrophobic, open MRI scanners are less threatening. Health maintenance organizations and managed care companies sometimes try not to cover some of these tests, but if they are essential, your doctor should always try to convince the company of their importance, and we recommend that you have the test if your doctor suggests it, even if it is not covered.

Electroencephalography (EEG), during which many wires are attached to the scalp, can be useful when evaluating headache patients whose histories include fainting, loss of consciousness, seizures, head trauma, or dizziness. The purpose is to look for evidence of a seizure disorder.

The most important part of your evaluation is the history that your doctor obtains from you. It alone can point to an accurate tentative diagnosis that can be confirmed by appropriate examination and, if necessary, testing. It is wise to prepare

Figure 5-2: Patient awaiting scanning by computed tomography (CT).

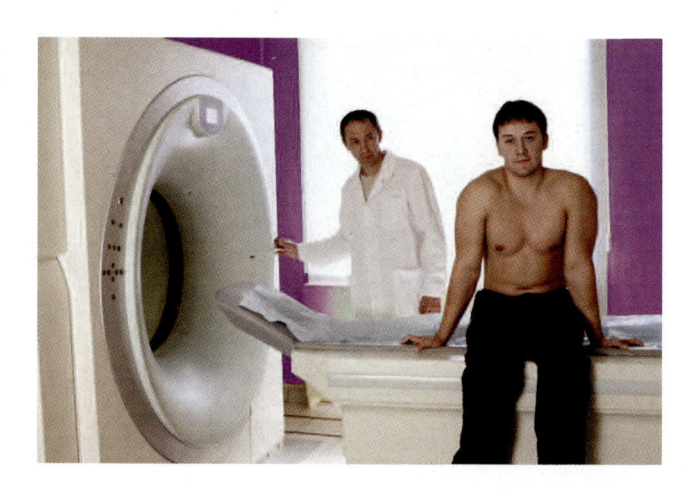

your history in advance by writing down all of your symptoms, the tests you have had, and the medications you have tried, with doses and how long you tried them. Put down if the medicine worked or not, if you experienced any side effects, what they were, and what your highest dose of the medicine was. Bring in headache calendars or diaries that you have kept (see Chapter 3), lists of medications, and reports of tests. Be sure to tell your doctor about the impact that your headaches have on your life. If there are times that, because of your headaches, you are unable to work, go to school, do household chores, or participate in family and social activities—or can only do these activities at a decreased level of effectiveness— discuss these issues with your doctor early in your visit. Most of the time, if the history and examination are complete and detailed at the first visit, a treatment plan can be begun immediately.

CONCERNS WITH DAILY HEADACHE

If your headaches occur daily or at least 15 days per month, that is, more often than not, be sure to let your doctor know this crucial fact. And if the headaches have recently changed pattern, that may be most important of all.

As noted in Chapter 4, there are multiple causes of and associations with daily headache. Specifically, a doctor will need to determine that a patient truly has *chronic* daily headache, that is, that the daily headache is of at least 3 months' duration. With the sudden, acute onset of daily headache, concerns rise about the possibility of bleeding into the head or an infection in or near the brain, and an imaging study and spinal tap often become necessary.

A spinal tap (lumbar puncture) may also be indicated if your headaches are severe and are associated with a stiff neck, fever, vomiting, and signs of either increased or decreased pressure in the brain. The most important abnormal findings from a spinal tap are evidence of bleeding, infection, or increased or decreased spinal fluid pressure, and all of these can be associated with the sudden onset of daily headache, or any headache.

When the onset of daily headache is acute but no cause is found, then the likely diagnosis becomes new daily persistent headache (NDPH) (see Chapter 4).

Because certain conditions that can be treated are strongly associated with daily headache, your doctor will look for these problems. As noted previously, they include abnormal thyroid disease, viral infections, Lyme disease (depending on where you live), stressful life events, frequency of medication use, caffeine intake, snoring, and obesity. There is a hope that attending to these problems can help prevent or treat daily headache.

HIGH- AND LOW-PRESSURE DAILY HEADACHES

Other causes of daily headache may be found when there are specific symptoms that a patient notices. For example, if the daily headaches go away when the patient is lying down but come on and worsen upon arising, there is a possibility of a leak of the cerebrospinal fluid from around the brain or spinal cord. Leaks can occur after trauma, anesthetic procedures, spinal taps, or surgery, but sometimes people with these leaks do not remember a causative event.

A common circumstance for a low-pressure positional daily headache is after an epidural anesthetic is placed for a birth, but in that circumstance, the daily headache will have been present for days, not months.

When a leak is suspected and the daily positional headache is of long standing, MRI with contrast dye is ordered, because in this study the contrast dye accumulates in the meninges or coverings of the brain in a highly characteristic way. A spinal tap may be performed to see if the pressure is low, and to introduce a special dye to look for the leak. If low-pressure daily headache is confirmed, the headache will sometimes respond to a procedure called a blood patch. This involves taking blood from the vein of the patient with the headache, and injecting it around the spinal column. Usually, an anesthesiologist performs the blood patch, which can often resolve the positional headache promptly, especially if the headache is of recent origin.

Blood patches work well when someone develops a low-pressure headache after an epidural, but may not work for a long-standing leak. In that circumstance, a series of imaging studies may be necessary to find the leak, and then a surgical procedure can be undertaken to fix the leak and resolve the daily headache.

High cerebrospinal fluid pressure can be another cause of daily headache. As a secondary chronic daily headache, it is called "idiopathic intracranial hypertension" but is commonly referred to as "pseudotumor cerebri." In this condition, some blockage prevents the normal cerebrospinal fluid circulation from functioning, and the fluid builds up, resulting in daily headache. In addition, the fluid can put pressure on the optic nerve, causing visual disturbance and even blindness if not diagnosed and treated properly. Pseudotumor occurs more commonly in obese younger or middle-aged women, and may be associated with intake of certain vitamins and antibiotics. The diagnosis always requires a spinal tap to check the cerebrospinal fluid pressure, and a careful eye exam by an ophthalmologist. Treatment can involve diuretics, steroids, or even a surgical procedure to divert the fluid.

Recognition of low or high cerebrospinal fluid conditions can be crucial in treating secondary daily headaches.

SINUS DISEASE

Many people think that sinus disease is a common cause of their daily headaches, but it is not. Headache is a *minor* feature of acute sinus infection, and occurs rarely. Headache is not usually a feature of chronic sinus disease. Migraine is commonly associated with red eyes, tearing, nasal stuffiness, postnasal drip, and congestion, as the parts of the brain that cause migraine also cause these phenomena. The term *sinus headache* was invented by advertisers to sell decongestants and over-the-counter antihistamines. In fact, ear, nose, and throat doctors do not recognize "sinus headaches" in their list of diagnoses. People commonly mistake migraines for "sinus headaches," and a study in 2004 of close to 3,000 people with either self-diagnosed or doctor-diagnosed "sinus headaches" found that around 90% of these headaches were migraine, while only 8 patients out of 2,991 people evaluated with "sinus headaches" had acute sinus infections. Thus, disabling headaches that last for 1 to 3 days, that occur several times per month, and that are associated with weather triggers, nasal stuffiness, clear drainage, tearing eyes, or postnasal drip are usually migraine.

Acute sinusitis is generally associated with fever, red-hot skin over the involved sinus, and a yellow-green, bad-tasting or -smelling discharge from the nostrils and back of the throat. Any headache associated with fever or infection must be treated immediately as an emergency. A severe acute sinus problem may trigger a typical migraine attack (Figure 5-3).

There are rare forms of sinusitis that can cause very serious headaches and can be life-threatening. These infections usually cause a change in headache pattern and a lack of response to previously effective treatment, which should always prompt a consult with a doctor. One such type is called sphenoid sinusitis, and it is diagnosed by CT or MRI of the sinuses.

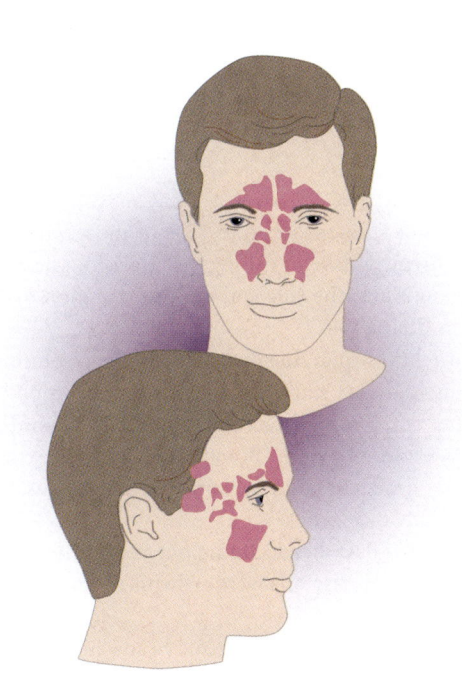

Figure 5-3: Diagram of sinuses in the head and face.

Chronic sinusitis is not a cause of chronic daily headaches. This remarkable fact, validated by the International Headache Society, should reassure those with daily headaches and help them look for other causes for their headaches or start treatment for one of the primary daily headache disorders, such as chronic migraine.

There is a rare cause of daily headache related to the sinuses that may be difficult to diagnose. This occurs when a small bone sticks into a part of the sinuses, and is called contact point headache. It is very rare, and those with this disorder have one-sided headache that must be distinguished from hemicrania continua (see Chapter 3).

BRAIN TUMOR

Brain tumors can cause daily headache, and the usual clue to the presence of a tumor is a change in the pattern of headaches. Thus, if someone has never had headaches, and develops daily headache, or if someone with headaches in discrete (separate) episodes develops daily headache, an imaging study is usually done to rule out a tumor. In people with migraine, the brain-tumor headache usually resembles chronic migraine, while in people with tension-type headache, the brain-tumor headache resembles chronic tension-type headache, but there is no "typical" brain-tumor headache. The most important clues for when to look for a tumor are the change in headache pattern and the development of daily headache. The previous description of brain-tumor headaches as usually present in the morning turns out to be unreliable. There are a few types of brain tumors in which headaches worsen with changes in head position; with that symptom, urgent consultation with a doctor is necessary.

NECK PAIN

Neck pain is frequent during migraine, present in up to 75% of those who suffer from migraine attacks, usually occurring before or during the attack, but occasionally after the pain is gone. Neck pain is also the rule and not the exception in daily headache, as has been described in Chapter 4.

Treatment of neck pain often relieves migraine and helps in the resolution of daily headache. For example, many patients state that they benefit from physical therapy, massage, osteopathic and other spinal manipulation, trigger point and nerve injections, and botulinum neurotoxin type A (Botox) injections. These interventions appear to help the primary headaches, but occasionally the neck itself has an abnormality that is a cause for daily headaches.

Neck problems as a primary cause of daily headache are not as common as once thought. It is relatively rare for a herniated disc or severe arthritis to cause chronic daily headache, and often difficult to diagnose.

There is a secondary daily headache, called cervicogenic headache, which can be a form of daily headache. In this headache, daily pain usually stays on one side of the neck, radiating up the back of the head to the eye, but remains on that side and does not switch sides. This is referred to as "side-locked pain." Neck positions can trigger or worsen the headache, which does not resemble migraine. Before considering the diagnosis of cervicogenic headache, a headache specialist will first treat for hemicrania continua with a trial of the medication indomethacin (see Chapter 3). If the neck-to-head side-locked pain does not respond to indomethacin, cervicogenic headache becomes a possibility.

In this circumstance, injections into the spine in the upper cervical region temporarily resolve the pain completely, and occasionally surgery can reproduce the relief of the injections. However, as noted, true cervicogenic headache is rare, while primary chronic daily headache with neck pain is relatively common.

The important fact to remember is that neck pain with daily headache is usually not a sign of an underlying neck problem, and that the types of treatments listed above, combined with the usual medications for chronic daily headache, are often both helpful and reassuring.

EYE-RELATED HEADACHE

Eye strain is not a common cause of chronic or recurrent headache. Headaches due to eye strain are generally mild and are felt in the forehead or in the eyes themselves. The pain is absent on awakening and worsens when the eyes are used for prolonged periods. Children with headaches are usually checked early for eye problems, which in fact are seldom found.

Glaucoma (increased pressure within the eye) may cause a headache that mimics a bad migraine or tension-type headache, or it may cause severe pain in and around the eye or in the forehead. If you notice changes in your vision, especially if you see halos around lights, accompanied by pain and other symptoms, consult an eye doctor at once.

TEMPOROMANDIBULAR JOINT DYSFUNCTION

The temporomandibular joint (TMJ) is located just in front of the ear, where the jaw meets the skull. Problems within the TMJ may cause ear or jaw pain, ringing in the ears, clicking in the joint, or pain (headache) in the area where the hinges of the jaw meet the upper face. Many patients with daily headaches have been misdiagnosed as having TMJ problems and have undergone major surgical reconstruction of the joint without experiencing any relief of their pain. Most "TMJ headaches" are actually migraine, muscle pain (called myofascial pain syndrome), or chronic daily headache. Some patients do grind their teeth at night and have sore jaw muscles, which can be a cause of early-morning headache but rarely causes significant daily headache. It can be treated with a variety of therapies, including botulinum neurotoxin type-A injections.

POST-TRAUMATIC HEADACHES

Post-traumatic headaches are caused by injury to the head or neck and may develop after what seems to be only a minor injury. The headaches usually begin within 24 hours to one week after the injury. Generally, daily post-traumatic headaches occur on both sides of the head, are constant, are mild to moderate in intensity, and can continue for months or years.

The great majority of people who suffer a head or neck injury in an automobile accident or strike their heads on a low beam have a daily headache for 48 hours to a few weeks. Sometimes the headaches become severe or even incapacitating, lasting for months or years, and they may resemble migraine at times. Patients with post-traumatic daily headache may be thought to be exaggerating their pain or malingering, but in our experience these patients have a debilitating disorder that may destroy the fabric of their lives and seriously impair their ability to function for years.

Some patients with post-traumatic daily headache also develop post-concussion syndrome and experience impaired concentration, memory, and sleep, as well as irritability, decreased energy and interests, depression, inability to perform sexually, personality changes, and decreased ability to handle even simple tasks.

The new onset of severe daily headache after trauma is always cause for concern, with bleeding in or over the top of the brain a serious consideration. For this reason, imaging studies are almost always performed after head and neck trauma in patients with daily headache.

In those with more persistent post-traumatic daily headaches, diagnostic tests such as scans of the brain or the cervical spine and electroencephalography (EEGs) usually fail to reveal abnormalities. However, the injury may have caused microscopic bleeding or tearing and damage to nerve fibers in the brain, brainstem, and spine, as well as metabolic changes. This damage, difficult to document, may disrupt the delicate balance of the chemical messengers that control pain.

Many patients develop post-traumatic headache as a result of whiplash (a neck injury) after a car accident in which they were "rear-ended." In this type of injury, the neck hyper-extends backwards and then snaps too far forwards, injuring muscles and ligaments. Sometimes patients do not even strike their head but have only this extension-flexion injury as the cause of their pain. The degree of head trauma does not necessarily correlate with the degree of pain intensity or disability. Pre-existing migraine or tension-type headache may worsen or begin after this kind of injury. Once again, treatments to the neck such as those described in the Neck section above, behavioral treatments such as relaxation therapies and biofeedback, along with anti-migraine medications and avoidance of overuse of analgesics, all can be helpful.

6

Treatment

Headache treatment can be broadly divided into two main categories: acute and preventive. For each of these categories, both pharmacologic and non-pharmacologic therapeutic modalities are available. The *preventive* treatments are used to prevent or decrease the frequency of a patient's headache. In addition, sometimes they shorten headache duration, decrease the intensity, and make acute-care medication work better. The *acute* treatments are used to abort or decrease a headache attack that is already in progress.

Preventive treatments are taken on a daily basis to reduce headache frequency. However, when taking acute medications, the frequent use of these treatments can actually lead to *worsening* of your headaches, as described earlier. Understanding this paradoxical effect, where more is not necessarily better, is essential for prevention and control of chronic daily headache.

The number of days during the week that acute treatments are used is more important than the number of doses that are taken on any given day. Acute medications of any type should not be used more than 2 or, at most, 3 days out of each week. Patients should think of all the acute treatment options and regard them as if they were one medication. Some doctors advise their patients to think of all their acute medicines as "medicine X" and to use this medication X less than 3 days per week and less than 10 days per month, to avoid medication overuse headaches.

In patients suffering from chronic daily headache, the only method of achieving this limited use of acute medication is to use a preventive approach. This forms the foundation of care for chronic daily headache. This approach is very different for the average headache patient whose headache occurs less frequently and in whom the acute treatments may be sufficient. For example, patients who have only two to three headache episodes per month may be managed with acute treatment options only. The only exception is infrequent headaches that last so long or cause so much disability that the patient needs preventive therapy.

PHARMACOLOGIC TREATMENTS

Preventive medications have been studied in patients with episodic migraine, not chronic migraine. Those that have been approved by the FDA for migraine prevention include two beta blockers—propranolol (Inderal) and timolol (Blocadren)—and two epilepsy medications—divalproex sodium (Depakote) and topiramate (Topamax). In addition, the tricyclic antidepressants such as amitriptyline (Elavil), although not FDA approved for migraine prevention, have shown significant benefit in double-blind placebo-controlled studies. Published data from clinical trials support the above medications as having the best efficacy and fewest side effects in terms of migraine prevention. Several other classes of medications are used off label to prevent migraine. There are far fewer studies of preventive medications in patients with chronic migraine than there are for episodic migraine.

Preventive Prescription Medications

The preventive prescription medications that have been extensively studied in patients with chronic daily headache are

- Topiramate (Topamax)
- Tizanidine (Zanaflex)
- Gabapentin (Neurontin)
- Fluoxetine (Prozac)
- Amitriptyline (Elavil)
- Botulinum toxin type A (Botox).

This group of medications works at various nerve receptors in the brain that may be either overactive or underactive in the patient with chronic migraine. The ideal site for medications to act as preventive agents in chronic migraine has not been established as yet, and you will note that the following medications have multiple sites at which they work on brain pathways. Recent work by Dr. Sheena Aurora shows that patients with chronic migraine have difficulty in dealing with excitation in the brain and that the use of these preventive medications might restore their ability to suppress it and thus prevent the cascade that leads to a migraine attack. It is thought that one of the first events in a migraine attack is the start of an abnormal electrical activity in the back of the brain called cortical spreading depression (see Chapter 4). Dr. Michael Moskowitz at Harvard has demonstrated that most effective migraine preventive medications decrease the chance of this "spreading depression" from forming.

Tizanidine (Zanaflex) prevents the release of norepinephrine in the lowest part of the brain (the brainstem) and in the peripheral nerves, which results in muscle relaxation and blocking of pain. Tizanidine is started at 2 mg per day and may be slowly increased up to 8 mg three times per day in chronic migraine patients. The biggest problem with too high a dose is drowsiness. Other side effects include dizziness, dry mouth, and weight loss.

Gabapentin (Neurontin) binds to small openings on the ends of nerve fibers, called calcium channels, and modulates their firing rates. This medication was originally approved for prevention of seizures in epileptic patients. In headache patients, gabapentin has been used in doses of 2,400 mg per day and has been shown to reduce the number of migraine days over the course of a month. The side effects that patients have reported with gabapentin include dizziness, drowsiness, unsteadiness on their feet, and nausea. Pregabalin (Lyrica) is similar to gabapentin and is presently being studied in patients with different types of migraine.

Topiramate is another medication originally used for epilepsy that works by blocking both sodium and calcium channels on the nerve cells in the brain. This blocking results in stabilizing the irritability in the nerve cells, which may prevent the cortical spreading depression that initiates some migraine attacks. In addition, topiramate increases the levels of an inhibitor in the brain called gamma-aminobutyric acid (GABA) and also blocks glutamate, which excites the brain. Topiramate was carefully studied in two large clinical trials, and 100 or 200 mg per day led to a significant reduction in the number of migraine days experienced by patients with episodic migraine. In another study it was found to help in chronic migraine. The main side effects that have been noted include tingling in the hands and feet (paresthesias), weight loss, and difficulty with finding words or remembering things. In rare cases, it caused kidney stones or an increase in pressure in the eyes, like glaucoma. If eye pain or visual problems occur with use of topiramate, patients should immediately have their eye pressures (tonometry) checked. Simply stopping the drug and taking some eye drops prevents further problems.

Fluoxetine (Prozac) is a type of antidepressant called a selective serotonin reuptake inhibitor (SSRI). This medication increases the amount of serotonin available at the nerve synapses in the brain, and results in a decrease in the number of available serotonin receptors. This will often improve mood and as a result may have an effect on reducing headache. Most doctors prefer to use this type of medication only for depression and anxiety and not for migraine. It can be tried in patients with chronic migraine in doses up to 40 mg per day. The side effects include fatigue, restlessness, insomnia, stomach pain, and blurred vision. More problematic possible side effects are a worsening of migraine, and sexual complaints such as difficulty having an orgasm.

Amitriptyline (Elavil) is another antidepressant that decreases serotonin receptors, increases the amount of serotonin available at the synapse, and also enhances the internal action of the opioid (analgesic) receptors. This medication has also shown benefit in patients with chronic tension-type headaches, which is a type of chronic daily headache. Side effects reported for amitriptyline include weight gain, constipation, palpitations, dry mouth, drowsiness, dizziness, fatigue, and confusion, especially in older patients.

A listing of preventive and acute-care medications—Category I medications for headache prevention, nonsteroidal anti-inflammatory drugs (NSAIDs), preventive anti-epilepsy and antidepressant medications, and triptans—is located at the end of this chapter, in Tables 6-1 to 6-5.

Other categories of medication that have been tried for preventing chronic migraine include calcium channel blockers, certain serotonin blockers, angiotensin-converting enzyme (ACE) inhibitors (used for blood pressure control); and angiotensin receptor blockers (also used for blood pressure control). Recently, a drug used to combat the symptoms of Alzheimer's disease, called memantine (Namenda), which blocks a receptor called the NMDA receptor, has been tried in migraine. It seems to work in some patients and does not have any severe side effects.

Botulinum toxin type A (Botox) has been extensively studied in patients with chronic migraine. Botulinum toxin is a chemical that is an established treatment for several neurologic and muscular disorders, including torticollis (in which the head turns involuntarily to one direction), stroke, cerebral palsy, severe sweating, and even facial wrinkles. It is derived from a bacterium called *Clostridium botulinum*. This toxin is associated with botulism, a form of food poisoning caused by eating improperly preserved food that has been contaminated with the *Clostridium botulinum* bacteria. (A patient would not develop botulism or food poisoning unless unusually large amounts of this toxin were swallowed. The amounts that are used therapeutically in the form of Botox consist of very small doses that cannot produce botulism.) Only two of the seven types of botulinum found in nature have been made into medications: type A, Botox, and type B, Myobloc. The most common medical use of botulinum toxin is to inject it into overactive muscles to produce muscle relaxation. The relaxation results as the botulinum toxin blocks the signal from the nerve to the muscle fiber. This prevents the muscles from contracting and has been an effective treatment for many overactive muscle spasm conditions. Similarly, botulinum toxin may block sensory nerve endings that are carrying pain information to the brain in the form of several chemicals. It is thought that Botox blocks glutamate, calcitonin gene-related peptide (CGRP) (see Chapter 4), and Substance P, all of which increase pain signals in peripheral nerves. This is the presumed mechanism of action in chronic migraine, where the botulinum toxin is injected around branches of the trigeminal nerve that carry sensation from the face and scalp regions (Figure 6-1).

Botulinum toxin has now been studied in more than 1,000 patients with chronic daily headache. Results from these trials suggest that this treatment may reduce the severity and frequency of headaches. The patients who appear to respond best to botulinum toxin are those who have headaches on more than 15 days per month and in whom the headaches are described as "imploding." This is a type of headache where the pain feels as if it is coming from outside of the head inwards. Examples of this would be a clamp or vice crushing the head, or feeling as if spikes are being driven into the head. Patients with eye pain also appear to be responders to this type of medication, whereas those that describe their pain as "exploding," or coming from the inside out, tend to be non-responders. The exploding type of headache may be described as the head feeling as if it is splitting open or feeling as if there is a need to drill a hole into the skull to relieve internal pressure.

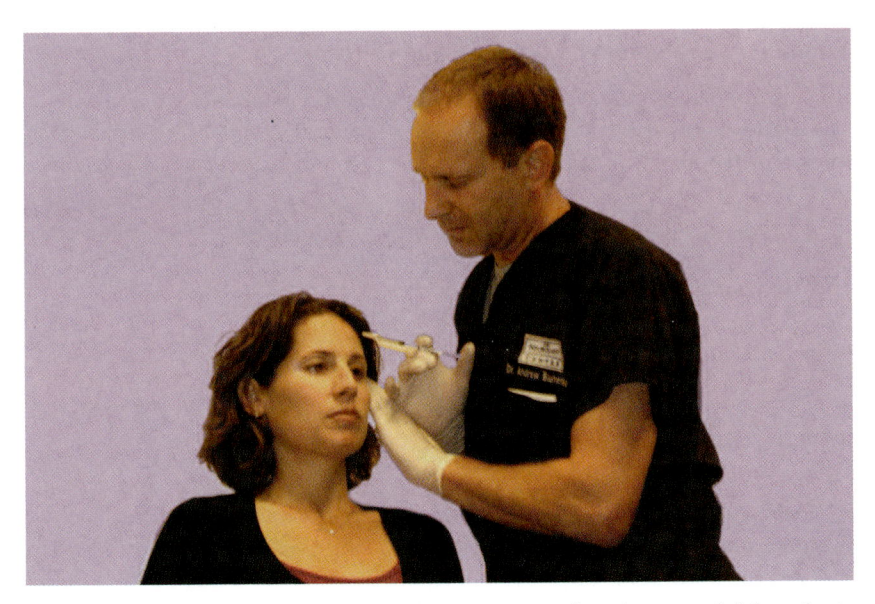

Figure 6-1: Injection of botulinum toxin to block sensory nerve endings that carry pain information to the brain.

The treatment of chronic migraine with botulinum toxin (Botox) involves injections of very small amounts of this medication into the muscles of the head and neck region close to the nerve endings (mainly the trigeminal nerve endings). This is achieved with a small needle, which is usually well tolerated, and the procedure can be done in minutes with minimal recovery time. No anesthesia or hospitalization is required, and patients leave the office shortly after the procedure. The effects take a few days to be noticed and usually increase over weeks to months. Botulinum toxin injections are not a cure for migraine, and frequently patients require repeat injections every 3 to 4 months, at least initially. Over time the treatments may become less frequent.

Botulinum toxin is considered a safe medication that has been used worldwide for multiple conditions, not only cosmetically but for many medical problems since 1989. Side effects are generally related to the injection technique. The injection can cause pain and bruising, and there is also a small risk of infection at the injection site. If too much medication is injected into the neck region, it could produce neck muscle weakness or difficulty swallowing. Injections around the eyes may lead to drooping of the eyelid or of the eyebrow. In general, side effects are short-lived and mild, usually resolving over weeks. One of the major benefits of botulinum toxin is that it is locally acting and thus has no systemic effects of any significance. The beneficial effects last for 3 to 4 months, and in many cases there is no longer any need to take a daily oral preventive medication.

Vitamins, Supplements, Minerals, and Herbs

Patients are often resistant to using daily preventive medications due to concerns about side effects. However, they are often willing to use "natural" agents, which include vitamins, minerals, supplements, and herbs. The most common agents utilized include:

- *Petasites hybridus* (butterbur)
- Magnesium
- Riboflavin
- Coenzyme Q10
- Melatonin
- Feverfew.

These products are not FDA approved and there is a lack of industrial standardization with respect to purity and content.

Petasites hybridus (Butterbur) (for which we prefer the brand name Petadolex) is a root extract of the Petasites plant. Doses of 50 mg of Petadolex three times a day may be used to reduce the number of migraine attacks. The main side effect noted with use of Petadolex was burping. To date, Petadolex is the best safety-tested herbal supplement of the headache treatments currently available.

Feverfew (*Tanacetum parthenium*) is derived from dried chrysanthemum leaves and has two potential active ingredients. These are melatonin and parthenolide. Current studies do not support feverfew as a highly recommended therapy for migraine. Side effects include sore mouth, sore tongue and lips, loss of taste, and gastrointestinal upset.

Magnesium supplements are thought to reduce migraine attacks, as ionized magnesium levels tend to be low in the blood of some migraine patients. The best formulation of magnesium has not been established. Most headache specialists suggest 400 to 800 mg of chelated magnesium per day. The side effects from magnesium are dose related and mainly involve diarrhea. If this occurs, a different salt of magnesium should be tried at a lower dose.

The use of *riboflavin* (vitamin B_2) in headache prevention has been investigated in only a couple of studies. Dosing probably requires at least 400 mg per day. However, one study showed benefit with only 25 mg of vitamin B_2 per day. In order to achieve a dose of 400 mg of vitamin B_2 per day, it is not recommended to take vitamin B_2 as part of a multivitamin, but rather to take 4 tablets of 100 mg vitamin B_2 per day.

Coenzyme Q10 at 300 mg per day has been reported in a single study to reduce migraine frequency.

Melatonin was studied in Brazil in an open trial in migraine patients, and 3 mg was shown to decrease migraine frequency. It may also provide benefit in headache types that are responsive to indomethacin (Indocin). Generally we recommend doses of 3 mg of melatonin three times a day. Many patients prefer to take them all at night as they induce sleep. Melatonin levels may in addition be low in cluster-type headaches, and in this population taking doses of 15 mg per day may be helpful.

Not all vitamins are beneficial for headache treatment. Some can worsen headaches, particularly niacin (vitamin B_1) and vitamin A.

NON-PHARMACOLOGIC MODALITIES

Non-pharmacologic treatments for chronic daily headache include:

- Exercise
- Weight loss
- Physical therapy
- Massage
- Acupuncture
- Chiropractic treatment
- Dental splints
- Nerve stimulators
- Magnetic devices

Frequent aerobic exercise may provide a true benefit and can promote weight loss. Obesity has been linked to the development of chronic daily headache, and thus weight reduction is important. Furthermore, endorphins, which are the body's own pain-relieving chemicals, are released during exercise and may reduce pain and stress. Physical therapy for neck pain may be helpful if it includes massage and gentle stretching exercises. Yoga techniques coupling physical exercise with breathing and relaxation as well as meditation have been shown to have positive effects in chronic pain conditions. In headache patients, yoga should include relaxation-focused postures and exclude vigorous bending activities. Exercises that involve straining efforts, such as heavy weightlifting, should be avoided.

Head and neck posture plays an important role in headache, particularly in tension-type headache, which may be present in some patients with frequent headaches. Forward head posture has been associated with painful trigger points in the neck and shoulder muscles. These trigger points have a taut band of skeletal muscle that is painful when compressed or stretched, and this gives rise to a referral pattern of pain that can include headache (Figure 6-2). Physical therapy aimed at improving head and neck posture may be helpful. The key therapy modalities involve pectoral (chest) muscle stretching, and exercises focused on improving the strength and bulk of the muscles between the shoulderblades, particularly the rhomboids and lower trapezius muscles.

Dental splints are frequently prescribed by dentists to help manage patients with headaches. At present, there is one dental splint that is FDA approved for the prevention of migraine headache, the nociceptive trigeminal inhibition (NTI) system. This is a splint that is custom made to fit over the incisors (the upper and lower center teeth) and prevents them from coming into contact. By keeping the upper and lower dentition separate, the patient is unable to clench the jaw. Clenching usually activates the temporalis muscles over the temples and masseter muscles of the cheeks, which send pain information to the trigeminal nerve. By limiting the activi-

Figure 6-2: Incorrect and correct posture. Excessive "tightness" in the upper chest and shoulder and a forward head position commonly result in headaches and in pain to the shoulders, neck, and upper back. Correct posture is shown at right.

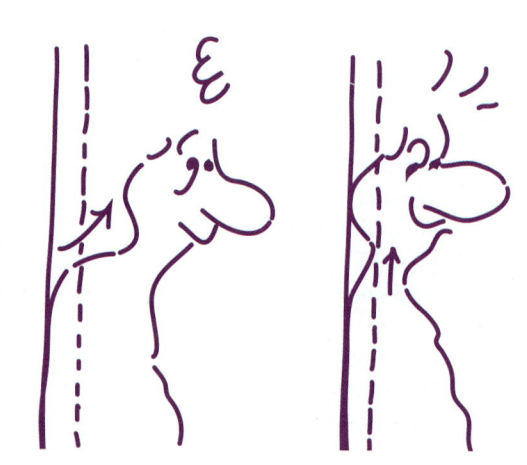

Chapter 6 Treatment   **47**

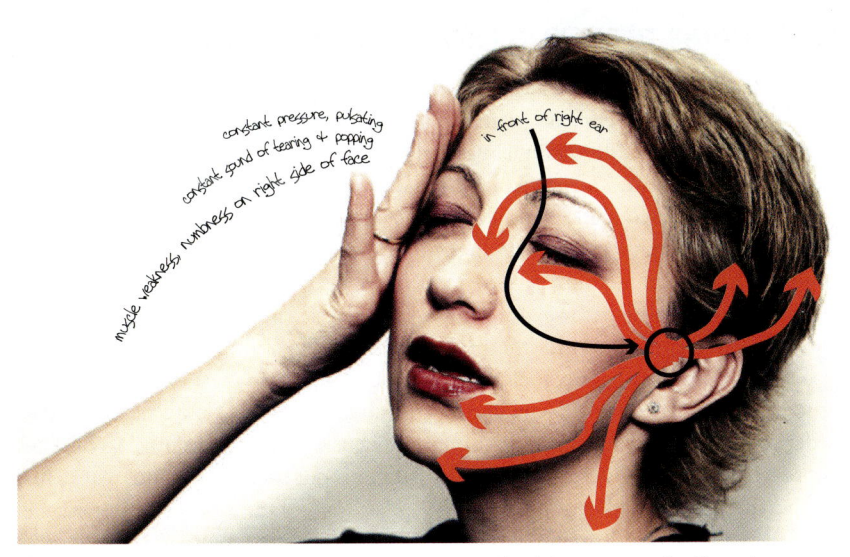

Figure 6-3: This drawing (adapted from one done by a patient) demonstrates the discomfort present over the temporomandibular joint (TMJ) with radiation to the face and head. Even though the patient has no medical background, by focusing on her pain she was able to outline branches of the trigeminal nerve (the main pain-sensing nerve of the face and head).

ty in these muscles, this splint may in fact be able to reduce trigeminal nerve activity and eliminate one of the triggers for headaches (Figure 6-3).

Acupuncture and *chiropractic treatment* have very little published data to support their use in the management of chronic daily headache. We do not like our patients over age 35 to have any manipulation of the neck, as this can cause injury to the major blood vessels carrying blood to the brain. Better-designed studies are needed to further investigate these treatments.

Some patients have received benefit from *local anesthetic injections* into the greater occipital nerve in the back of the head, and many studies have been done on this technique.

Research is ongoing for the use of *occipital nerve stimulators* and *magnetic devices*. The occipital nerve stimulator is a device implanted just under the skin in the area of the occipital nerves at the back of the head. It works by sending electrical pulses through those nerves into the brainstem to block pain signals. This is currently being investigated for patients who have failed to respond to all the other treatment modalities listed above. Magnetic stimulators are handheld devices used to abort the acute migraine attack. At present, studies on these devices are in the early exploratory stage. We think this may be particularly important in patients who are overusing acute oral medications, as the aggravating factor of medication overuse can be avoided with this device. These treatments may provide new insights and offer hope for those patients whose symptoms have not improved with the current available therapies.

MEDICATIONS TO AVOID IN CHRONIC DAILY HEADACHE

Excessive use of *any acute medicine* in the treatment of severe headaches may result in a paradoxical increase in intensity and frequency of headaches in chronic headache sufferers. Additionally, abnormal pain can occur in response to prolonged use of acute medications, particularly opiates (eg, oxycodone and its long-acting form OxyContin; codeine; hydrocodone [Vicodin]; meperidine [Demerol]; and many others). Recently, structural changes in the nervous system caused by opiate exposure have been identified. These involve the nerve pathways that descend into the spinal cord. These pathways may in fact become sensitized, allowing patients to feel spontaneous pain and to interpret light touch as painful. These changes may also occur with non-opiate analgesics. As a result, the use of sustained opiate or other pain therapy for headache patients requires that the patient's headache disorder be refractory to progressive, comprehensive, and preventive treatment approaches that are undertaken while the patient is not overusing acute treatments.

Furthermore, medications used for *other conditions* can cause headache. Examples are the proton-pump inhibitors used to treat acid reflux, some blood pressure-lowering drugs, and others. All prescription and non-prescription medications should be carefully screened to assess whether headache is a potential side effect, and if this is the case a trial period without this treatment should be considered.

OPTIONS IN ACUTE TREATMENT

The most effective acute treatment should have the goal of achieving a headache-free state within 2 hours and having a sustained effect for at least 24 hours. This should lead to a limitation in the number of days that the acute medications are needed. In general, fast-acting triptans are ideal for this purpose. These are sumatriptan (Imitrex), eletriptan (Relpax), almotriptan (Axert), rizatriptan (Maxalt) and zolmitriptan (Zomig). These triptans should be taken early in the course of the migraine attack to optimize their effect. The two slower-acting triptans frovatriptan (Frova) and naratriptan (Amerge) can also be helpful, and may work quickly if taken early. We teach our patients to take their triptan once the headache becomes throbbing or is worsened by head movement. Ideally, they need to take their triptan before the head and scalp become sensitive to touch, which usually occurs 30 minutes to an hour into the migraine attack. This sensitivity to touch is termed "allodynia" and can be tested for by combing your hair, which instead of feeling pleasant will be uncomfortable during a migraine attack. Patients often report that, as their migraine progresses, they do not want anything to touch their head or scalp and they remove earrings and hair accessories. The short-acting triptans are more effective if taken at this early stage of the migraine than later in the attack. Ideally, these medications should also be limited to a maximum of 2 days per week. This requires the patient's careful recording of the medications used during the course of a week on a calendar.

Preliminary data supporting the use of long-acting triptans such as naratriptan (Amerge) on a daily basis for 3 to 6 months as a preventive option for intractable chronic migraine are emerging. This has been done only on an experimental basis. Using non-triptan medication, such as the nonsteroidal anti-inflammatories (naproxen, which in its off-the-shelf form is Aleve) or combination analgesics such as Fiorinal (butalbital combined with caffeine and aspirin) may be helpful, but is less likely to result in a pain-free state and as a result may lead to medication overuse. The key to this issue is to make sure that the use of the acute medication is not escalating while the headaches worsen. The use of the acute treatments is probably responsible for the deterioration.

PROPER USE OF PREVENTIVE TREATMENT OPTIONS

Preventive treatment modalities need to be used for at least a 6-month period once an effective medication is found. As a result, prior to initiating these treatments a process of shared decision making should be undertaken. The key to success in this process is that the physician should educate the patient about the treatment options, the efficacy data, and the side effects, and then a detailed discussion should take place with the patient to ensure buy-in to using the medication so that adequate patient compliance will be achieved. Co-morbidity (the presence of other medical problems) is an important factor to consider in choosing a medication. For example, studies have shown an association between migraine, major depression, and anxiety disorders including panic attacks, obsessive-compulsive disorder, and generalized anxiety.

Medications that may help treat both headache and these related conditions include tricyclic antidepressants like amitriptyline (Elavil), and this may be an ideal option in the patient who has both conditions. However, we often use these antidepressants in patients with chronic migraine who are not depressed, and the fact that these are prescribed by your physician does not necessarily mean that he feels you are depressed. They can also help you sleep through the night.

Some patients have both chronic headache and high blood pressure, and several medications may treat both conditions—beta blockers like propranolol (Inderal) and angiotensin receptor blockers such as candasartan (Atacand).

For the patient in whom obesity is problematic, medication such as topiramate may be beneficial. In patients with epilepsy, anticonvulsants like topiramate or divalproex sodium would be appropriate choices. Ideally, patients should be managed with a single medication. However, often this is simply not feasible. We generally begin with a single treatment starting at a low dose and then gradually titrate (increase the dose), while simultaneously managing the side effects and trying to maximize the benefit of the treatment before adding a second agent. Often the first agent may result in only partial benefit, so combination approaches are used to work towards a headache-free state.

Interactions between different drugs need to be considered whenever more than one medication is used. Recently, the serotonin syndrome has been in the news. This is a reaction resulting from excessive serotonin activity. Its effects can range from mild to fatal. This rare condition has been reported when triptans are combined with selective serotonin reuptake inhibitors such as fluoxetine (Prozac) or selective serotonin-norepinephrine reuptake inhibitors such as duloxetine (Cymbalta). The serotonin syndrome includes tremor, weakness, clumsiness, somnolence, coma, brisk reflexes, and jerky eye movements. Patients who develop the full-blown syndrome will require hospitalization.

If all of the above modalities are tried adequately and the patient fails to respond, then the diagnosis needs to be reviewed. Other possible contributors to the headache disorder may be complicating management. For example, obstructive sleep apnea, which involves excessive daytime fatigue, loud snoring, and cessation of breathing for brief periods of time during sleep, can cause a daily headache. Rarely, more serious conditions may be present, such as sphenoid sinusitis, brain tumor, blood vessel blockage in the brain, change in spinal fluid pressure, or meningitis. A full neurologic examination and proper testing can rule out these conditions.

SUMMARY

Chronic headache can be managed using combinations of pharmacologic and non-pharmacologic treatment modalities. Patients need close supervision by their physicians and frequent follow-up visits to coordinate their care. Educating the patient about the underlying condition, the triggers that can worsen the headache disorder, and the expectations that they can hope to achieve with the medication are key to success.

Additional information in regard to patient education can be found at <www.theheadachecenter.com>, <www.headachenech.com>, and <www.hcop.com>.

Table 6.1: Category I* for Headache Prevention: Fewest Side Effects and Greatest Efficacy

Amitriptyline
Divalproex sodium
Propranolol
Timolol
Topiramate

*These are the main medications suggested for prevention by the American Headache Society.

Pregnancy category C,D (3rd trimester)

Use of all drugs listed in the tables in the following pages is not advised in pregnancy, with SSRIs and triptans the exception (pregnancy category C). Even SSRIs were indicated as causing persistent pulmonary hypertension in newborns and are not recommended.

Drugs considered acceptable in pregnancy by some physicians include acetaminophen, Fiorinal and opioids (not on a chronic basis). Your doctor may or may not want to use these drugs if you are pregnant.

Table 6.2: Nonsteroidal Anti-inflammatory Drugs Commonly Used for Chronic Daily Headache

Generic Name	Brand Names	Dose (mg)	Side Effects	Comments
Naproxen	Naprosyn	250, 375, 500	Can cause stomach ulcers, kidney problems, elevated blood pressure, and excessive bleeding	—
Naproxen sodium	Anaprox	275, 550	See under Naproxen	—
	Naprelan	375, 500		—
	Aleve	220		—
Diclofenac	Cataflam	25, 26, 75, 100	See above	—
	Voltaren			
	Voltaren-XR			
Indomethacin	Indocin	25, 50	See above, plus eye problems and occasional drowsiness	—
	Indocin SR	75 SR only		—
Etodolac	Lodine	200, 300, 400	Can cause stomach ulcers, kidney problems, elevated blood pressure, and excessive bleeding	—
	Lodine XL	400, 500, 600		—
Ibuprofen	Advil	200	See above	—
	Motrin	400, 600, 800		—
Fenoprofen	Nalfon	200, 300	See above	—
Ketoprofen	Orudis KT	12.5	See above	—
	Orudis	25, 50, 75		—
	Oruvail	100, 150, 200		—
Flurbiprofen	Ansaid	100	See above	—
Mefenamic acid	Ponstel	250	See above	—
Nabumetone	Relafen	500, 750	See above	—
Meclofenamate	Meclomen	100, 200	See above	—
Ketorolac	Toradol	10 pill, 30 or 60 mg ampoule for injection	See above, plus higher incidence of ulcers	Limited to max of 5 days use, 1st dose should be IV or IM then switch to oral
Celecoxib	Celebrex	100, 200	See above, but lower incidence of stomach problems	A new cyclo-oxygenase 2 (Cox-2) inhibitor

Table 6.3: Preventive Anti-epilepsy Drugs

None are for use by women who are or may be pregnant

Generic Name	Brand Name	Dosage Range (mg/day)	Side Effects
Divalproex sodium	Depakote	500 – 1,500	Drowsiness, hair loss, tremor, diarrhea, weight gain, foot swelling, inflammation of liver, bone marrow, or pancreas **Not for use in people with liver disease or in combination with barbiturates**
Gabapentin	Neurontin	600 – 2,700	Drowsiness, dizziness, weight gain
Topiramate	Topamax	45 – 200	Weight loss, confusion, kidney problems and stones, glaucoma, loss of sweating, tingling of arms and legs
Zonisamide	Zonegran	25 – 400	Weight loss, drowsiness, kidney problems and stones, tingling of arms and legs, lack of sweating
Tiagabine	Gabitril	8 – 48	Drowsiness, nausea
Pregabalin	Lyrica	150 - 600	Drowsiness, dizziness, peripheral edema, weight gain, xerostomia, tremor, myoclonus
Lamotrigine	Lamictal	100 - 200	Rash, nausea, Stevens Johnson Syndrome (SJS) associated with rapid dose escalation, starting dose of 25 mg recommended

Table 6.4: Antidepressants

Tricyclic Antidepressants

Generic Name	Brand Name
Amitriptyline	Elavil
Doxepin	Sinequan, Adapine
Nortriptyline	Pamelor
Desipramine	Norpramin
Trazodone	Desyrel
Imipramine	Tofranil
Amoxapine	Asendin
Protriptyline	Vivactil
Maprotiline	Ludiomil
Clomipramine	Anaframil

Selective Serotonin Reuptake Inhibitors

Generic Name	Brand Name
Citalopram	Celexa
Escitalopram	Lexapro
Fluoxetine	Prozac
Fluvoxamine	Luvox
Sertraline	Zoloft
Paroxetine	Paxil

Serotonin Norepinephrine Reuptake Inhibitors

Generic Name	Brand Name
Venlafaxine	Effexor
Duloxetine	Cymbalta

Miscellaneous

Generic Name	Brand Name
Bupropion	Wellbutrin
Mirtazapine	Remeron
Nefazodone	Serzone

Monoamine Oxidase Inhibitors

Generic Name	Brand Name
Phenelzine	Nardil
Isocarboxazid	Marplan
Tranylcypromine	Parnate

Table 6.5: Triptans

Generic Name	Brand Name	Form	Dose (mg)	Maximum Quantity in 24 H (mg)	Comes in Box of
Group I					
Sumatriptan	Imitrex*	Subcutaneous injection	6	12	2
		Tablet	25, 50, 100 (100 is best dose)	200/24 hours	9
		Nasal spray	5, 20 (20 is best starting dose)	40	6
Zolmitriptan	Zomig*	Tablet	2.5 5	10 10	6 (2.5 mg) 3 (5 mg)
	Zomig ZMT*	Melt	2.5 5	10 10	6 (2.5 mg) 3 (5 mg)
	Zomig*	Nasal spray	5	10	6 (5 mg)
Rizatriptan	Maxalt*	Tablet, melt	5, 10 (10 is best dose); 5 if on propranonol)	30 (15 if on propranonol)	12
Almotriptan	Axert*	Tablet	12.5	25	6
Eletriptan	Relpax*	Tablet	20, 40 (40 is best dose)	80	6
Naratriptan	Amerge**	Tablet	1, 2.5	5	9
Frovatriptan	Frova**	Tablet	2.5	7.5	9
Dihydroergotamine: Migranal nasal spray			4 sprays, totaling 2 mg		

Potential triptan side effects

Nuisance
Tingling of hands and fingers, flushing, paresthesia, warmth, chest and neck pressure, drowsiness or dizziness
Important to tell your doctor
Chest pain

*quick-acting; **slow-acting.

7

A Final Word

If you have reached this part of the book, we assume you have had frequent and severe headaches for much too long. You have been to many doctors and tried a variety of treatments. We understand your situation and you are not alone. Patients with chronic headache spend much of their day treating their pain and still suffering, while searching for answers and for more effective treatment.

Chronic daily headache was described as long ago as 350 years and the issue of medication overuse or rebound has been observed for nearly a century. Currently over 10 million people in the United States experience daily headache. They contribute greatly to the cost of disability in the US ($20 billion dollars per year) and of course experience much personal suffering and inability to function optimally. In fact, research tells us that the burden of illness is greater for chronic headache patients than for those with Parkinson's disease, multiple sclerosis, Alzheimer's disease and epilepsy combined! But since patients with chronic headache often suffer in silence, those around them may not know or understand.

We hope you find this book useful and that you have a better understanding of the types of headache you have and the available treatments. Chronic headache is rarely curable, but it is very amenable to treatment. With optimal therapy, your headaches should be fewer, milder, and shorter in duration. You should be able to do more and function better. Your best defense against continuing chronic headache is expert education about the problem and a sympathetic, knowledgeable headache specialist. Management of chronic daily headache presents a significant challenge for you and your caregivers. Although treatment may take time and may present various roadblocks, there is no need to despair. This is *not* a disorder that "you have to learn to live with." Rather, it is one that requires effective treatment so that you can live optimally.

Headache specialists now understand more clearly the causes of headache and we are better at diagnosing the types of chronic headache. There are a myriad of non-pharmacologic treatments, which include making some significant lifestyle changes, working with behavioral medicine experts to learn self-help techniques and minimize your triggers, and using a combination of the most effective daily preventive and acute-care medications. Special techniques like occipital nerve stimulation, deep brain stimulation, and botulinum toxin type-A injections, although not yet approved by the FDA, are helping many with chronic headache.

You have now learned that the overuse of acute-care medication ("medication-overuse headache") is one of the most significant causes of ongoing chronic headache. Mastering this problem may be difficult, but it is possible.

Some special points to remember are:

1. Opiates (narcotics) rarely help the pain of chronic headache and probably worsen it over time. Many alternatives are available.
2. Using acute-care medications (including off-the-shelf medications) more than 2 days a week often leads in the direction of rebound or medication overuse headache.
3. While daily preventive medications may bring results, you may need to be taking more than one prescription medication in addition to vitamins, minerals, supplements, and herbs that have been shown in studies to help headache.
4. More than one cup of coffee per day, or other sources of caffeine, may worsen your headache over time.
5. Your personal triggers must be avoided as best you can.

Remember, you are not alone. Many headache specialists like us have devoted their lives to research and treatment of chronic headache problems. There is probably a headache specialist near you. Also, there are many resources on line, such as:

- The American Council for Headache Education (ACHE): www.achenet.org
- The National Headache Foundation (NHF): <www.headaches.org>)
- Migraine Awareness Group: A National Understanding for Migraineurs (MAGNUM): <www.migraines.org>
- Teri Roberts (author and advocate for migraineurs, featured on MyMigraineConnection.com) at: <http://www.healthcentral.com/migraine>

Four of our sites are:

- The Headache Center in San Diego: <www.the-headachecenter.com>
- The New England Center for Headache in Stamford, Connecticut: <www.headachenech.com>
- The Headache Cooperative of New England: <www.hacoop.org>
- The Headache Cooperative of the Pacific: <www.hcop.com>.

In our experience, 85% of patients with chronic headache can obtain significant relief from ongoing, expert care. We hope you will become one of them.

Index

A
Abnormal sounds, 31f
ACE. *See* Angiotensin converting enzyme (ACE) inhibitors
Acupuncture, 47
Acute sinusitis, 35
Adapine, 53t
Advil, 51t
Aerobic exercise
 frequent, 46
Alcoholic beverages
 triggering migraine, 22–23, 24t
Aleve, 49, 51t
Almotriptan (Axert), 48, 54t
Amerge, 48, 49, 54t
Amitriptyline (Elavil), 7, 40, 42, 49, 50t, 53t
Amoxapine (Asendin), 53t
Anacin, 23, 26
 caffeine content of, 25t
Anaframil, 53t
Analgesics, 7
Anaprox, 51t
Anesthetic injections
 local, 47
Anesthetics
 epidural, 34
Angiotensin converting enzyme (ACE) inhibitors, 42
Angiotensin receptor blockers, 42
Ansaid, 51t
Anticonvulsant medications, 49
Antidepressant medications
 tricyclic, 53t
 triggering migraine, 23t
Anxiety, 1, 26
Arthritis, 27
Asendin, 53t
Aspartame
 triggering migraine, 23t, 24t
Aura
 and CSD, 19, 20
 with migraine, 11
 visual, 13
Aurora, Sheena, 41
Avocado
 triggering migraine, 24t
Axert, 48, 54t

B
Bacon
 triggering migraine, 24t
Baleat, Ray, 5–6
Bananas
 triggering migraine, 24t

Beer
 triggering migraine, 22
Bending over, 30
Beverages
 alcohol triggering migraine, 22–23
 caffeine content of cocoa, 25t
Bigal, Marcelo, 27
Biofeedback, 22
Blocadren, 40, 50t
Blood patches, 34
Blood pressure medications, 42, 48
 triggering migraine, 23t
Boes, Chris, 4, 7
Bologna
 triggering migraine, 24t
Botulinum neurotoxin type A (Botox), 22, 37, 40, 42–44, 43f
 for neck pain, 36
Bowel movement, 30
Brain
 anatomy of, 19f
 hyperexcitable, 18
 magnesium, 19
 migraine-prone, 18
 sensitive, 18
Brainstem, 19
Brain tumors
 causing daily headaches, 36
Bruits, 31f
Bupropion (Wellbutrin), 53t
Burstein, Rami, 21
Butalbital, 23, 49
 caffeine content of, 25t
Butterbur, 44

C
Cafergot, 23
Caffeine, 27t, 56
 in foods and drugs, 25t
 overuse headache, 26
 triggering migraine, 23, 24t, 25
Caffenism, 25
Calcitonin gene-related peptide (CGRP), 21, 43
Calcium channel blockers, 42
Calendar
 headache, 12, 13f
California Medical Clinic for Headache, 6
Canned figs
 triggering migraine, 24t
Capobianco, David, 4, 7
Cataflam, 51t
CAT scan. *See* Computed tomography (CAT scan)
CDH. *See* Chronic daily headache (CDH)
Celecoxib (Celebrex), 51t

Celexa, 53t
Central sensitization, 21
Cerebrospinal fluid pressure, 34
Cervicogenic headache, 36–37
CGRP. *See* Calcitonin gene-related peptide (CGRP)
Champagne
    triggering migraine, 22
Cheese
    triggering migraine, 23, 24t
Children
    parentified, 2
Chiropractic treatment, 47
Chocolate
    caffeine content of, 25t
    triggering migraine, 24t
Chronic daily headache (CDH)
    causes of, 20–21
    characteristics of, 9t
    classification of, 14
    description, 5
    impact, 1–2
    NSAIDs for, 51t
    prevalence, 3
Chronic headache
    diagnosis of, 8–9
Chronic migraine (CM), 14
    classification of, 14–15
    description, 5
    impact, 1–2
Chronic sinusitis, 36
Chronic tension-type headache (CTTH), 14
Circle of Willis, 4
Citalopram (Celexa), 53t
Clomipramine (Anaframil), 53t
Clostridium botulinum, 42
Cluster headache
    characteristics of, 9t
    classification of, 14
    diagnosis of, 8–9
CM. *See* Chronic migraine (CM)
Coca-Cola
    caffeine content of, 25t
Cocoa beverages
    caffeine content of, 25t
Codeine, 48
Coenzyme Q10, 44, 45
Coffee
    caffeine content of, 25t
Collier, James, 5
Computed tomography (CAT scan), 11, 32, 32f
Computer terminals, 27
Concentration, 2
Consultation
    of doctors, 29–30
Cortex, 19
Cortical spreading depression (CSD), 19–20
Coughing, 30
CSD. *See* Cortical spreading depression (CSD)
CTTH. *See* Chronic tension-type headache (CTTH)
Cymbalta, 50, 53t

D
Daily headache
    concerns with, 33
    risks for developing, 27t
Danger signals, 30
Darvon compound
    caffeine content of, 25t
Demerol, 48
Dental splints, 46–47
Depakote, 40, 49, 50t, 52t
Depression, 1, 26
Desipramine (Norpramin), 53t
Desyrel, 53t
Diary
    headache, 12, 30
Diclofenac (Cataflam, Voltaren), 51t
Dietary triggers, 24t
Diet Coke
    caffeine content of, 25t
Dihydroergotamine, 54t
Disability, 2, 55
Disk disease
    neck, 27
Divalproex sodium (Depakote), 40, 49, 50t, 52t
Doctors
    consultation of, 29–30
    discussions with patients, 11–12
    questions asked by, 31t
    role, 30
Double vision, 30
Doxepin (Sinequan, Adapine), 53t
Dr. Pepper
    caffeine content of, 25t
Duloxetine (Cymbalta), 50, 53t

E
Economic cost
    of headache, 2–3, 55
EEG. *See* Electroencephalography (EEG)
Effexor, 53t
Elavil, 7, 40, 42, 49, 50t, 53t
Electroencephalography (EEG), 32
Eletriptan (Relpax), 48, 54t
Endorphins, 46
Epidural anesthetics, 34
Equal (aspartame)
    triggering migraine, 23t, 24t
Escitalopram (Lexapro), 53t
Esgic
    caffeine content of, 25t
Etodolac (Lodine), 51t
Evil spirits, 4
Excedrin, 26
Excedrin Migraine, 23
    caffeine content of, 25t
Exercise, 30
Extra-strength Excedrin
    caffeine content of, 25t
Extremity weakness or numbness, 30
Eye-related headache, 37

Index

F
Family life, 2
Fatigue, 2
Fenoprofen (Nalfon), 51t
Fermented foods
   triggering migraine, 24t
Feverfew *(Tanacetum parthenium)*, 44, 45
Fifth cranial nerve, 20
Figs
   triggering migraine, 24t
Fioricet
   caffeine content of, 25t
Fiorinal (butalbital), 23, 49
   caffeine content of, 25t
Fluoxetine (Prozac), 40, 42, 50, 53t
Flurbiprofen (Ansaid), 51t
Foods
   triggering migraine, 22–23, 24t
France, 5
Frequent aerobic exercise, 46
Friedman, Arnold, 6
Frova, 48, 54t
Frovatriptan (Frova), 48, 54t

G
GABA. *See* Gamma-aminobutyric acid (GABA)
Gabapentin (Neurontin), 40, 41, 52t
Gabitril, 52t
Gamma-aminobutyric acid (GABA), 41
Genetics
   migraine, 18
Glaucoma, 37

H
Ham
   triggering migraine, 24t
Harvard Medical School, 21, 41
Harvey, William, 4–5
HC. *See* Hemicrania continua (HC)
Headache
   acute treatment options, 48–49
   causes and risk factors of, 17–28
   characteristics of, 9t
   classification of, 12–13
   diagnosis of, 8–16
   economic cost of, 2–3, 55
   epidemiology of, 1–3
   historical background, 4–7
   history, 8–9
   impact, 1–3
   non-pharmacologic modalities, 45–48
   pharmacologic treatment of, 40–41
   prevalence, 1–3
   prevention, 11
   preventive treatment of, 39, 49–50, 50t
   symptoms, 2
   treatment of, 11, 39–54
Headache calendar, 12, 13f
Headache diary, 12, 30
Head and neck posture, 46

Head-forward posture, 27
Head injury, 27t
Health-care provider
   consultation of, 29–30
   discussions with patients, 11–12
   questions asked by, 31t
   role, 30
Hemicrania continua (HC), 14
   classification of, 16
Herbs, 44–45
High- and low-pressure daily headaches, 33–34
HIV. *see* Human immunodeficiency virus (HIV)
Horton, Bayard, 6
Hot dogs
   triggering migraine, 24t
Human immunodeficiency virus (HIV), 30
Hydrocodone (Vicodin), 48
Hyperexcitable brain, 18
Hypertension
   idiopathic intracranial, 34
Hysteria, 5

I
Ibuprofen (Advil, Motrin), 51t
Idiopathic intracranial hypertension, 34
IHS. *See* International Headache Society (IHS)
Imipramine (Tofranil), 53t
Imitrex, 48, 54t
Inderal, 40, 50t
Indomethacin (Indocin), 45, 51t
Infections, 27t
Intermittent migraine, 2
International Headache Society (IHS), 14
Isocarboxazid (Marplan), 53t

J
Jaw
   tense, 27
Jobs, 2

K
Ketoprofen (Orudis, Oruvail), 51t
Ketorolac (Toradol), 51t
Kudrow, Lee, 6

L
Lamotrigine (Lamictal), 52t
Lenox, William, 6
Lexapro, 53t
Lipton, Richard, 2
Local anesthetic injections, 47
Lodine, 51t
Ludiomil, 53t
Lumbar puncture, 33
Lyme disease, 27, 27t, 32
Lyrica, 41, 52t

M
Magnesium, 44, 45
   brain, 19

Magnetic devices, 47–48
Magnetic resonance angiography (MRA), 11, 32
Magnetic resonance imaging (MRI scan), 11, 32
Magnetic resonance venography (MRV), 11
Maprotiline (Ludiomil), 53t
Marplan, 53t
Massage
  for neck pain, 36
Mathew, Ninan, 2
Maxalt, 48, 54t
Meats
  triggering migraine, 24t
Meclofenamate (Meclomen), 51t
Meclomen, 51t
Medication overuse headache (MOH)
  classification of, 15
Medications
  anticonvulsant, 49
  to avoid in chronic daily headache, 48
  blood pressure, 42
  overuse of, 7, 15, 27t
  prescription
    caffeine content of, 25t
  preventive
    headache calendars, 12
  preventive anti-epilepsy, 52t
  preventive prescription, 40–41
  triggering migraine, 23t
Mefenamic acid (Ponstel), 51t
Melatonin, 44, 45
Memantine (Namenda), 42
Memory, 2
Menstrual cycle
  triggering migraine, 22
Meperidine (Demerol), 48
MIDAS (Migraine Disability Assessment Scale)
  Questionnaire, 2
Migraine. *See also* Chronic migraine (CM)
  causes of, 18–19
  characteristics of, 9t
  diagnosis of, 8–9
  dietary triggers of, 24t
  genetics, 18
  intermittent, 2
  with or without aura, 12–13
  prevention of, 40
  transformed, 2
  triggers, 18, 22–23, 23t, 24f, 35, 37
Migraine Disability Assessment Scale (MIDAS)
  Questionnaire, 2
Migraine-prone brain, 18
Minerals, 44–45
Mirtazapine (Remeron), 53t
MOH. *See* Medication overuse headache (MOH)
Monoamine oxidase inhibitors, 53t
Monosodium glutamate (MSG)
  triggering migraine, 23t
Montefiore Headache Clinic, 6
Moskowitz, Michael, 41
Motrin, 51t

Mountain Dew
  caffeine content of, 25t
MRA. *See* Magnetic resonance angiography (MRA)
MRI scan. *See* Magnetic resonance imaging (MRI scan)
MRV. *See* Magnetic resonance venography (MRV)
MSG. *See* Monosodium glutamate (MSG)
Muscle-contraction headaches, 27
Myobloc, 42
Myofascial pain syndrome, 37

N
Nabumetone (Relafen), 51t
Nalfon, 51t
Namenda, 42
Naprelan, 51t
Naproxen (Naprosyn), 51t
Naproxen sodium (Anaprox, Naprelan, Aleve), 51t
Naratriptan (Amerge), 48, 49, 54t
Narcotics, 56
Nardil, 53t
NDPH. *See* New daily persistent headache (NDPH)
Neck, 27
  pain, 36–37
  posture, 46
Nefazodone (Serzone), 53t
Neurasthenia, 5
Neurological examination, 31f
Neurontin, 40, 41, 52t
New daily persistent headache (NDPH), 14, 33
  causes of, 22
  classification of, 16
New England Center for Headache, 7
Nitroglycerin
  triggering migraine, 23t
Nociceptive trigeminal inhibition (NTI) system, 46
No-Doz tablets
  caffeine content of, 25t
Nonsteroidal anti-inflammatory drugs (NSAIDs), 42, 51t
Norpramin, 53t
Nortriptyline (Pamelor), 53t
NP. *See* Nurse practitioner (NP)
NSAID. *See* Nonsteroidal anti-inflammatory drugs (NSAIDs)
NTI. *See* Nociceptive trigeminal inhibition (NTI) system
Nurse practitioner (NP), 12
Nutrasweet
  triggering migraine, 23t, 24t
Nuts
  triggering migraine, 24t

O
Obesity, 27t, 46
  causing headache, 27

Occipital nerve stimulators, 47
Off-the-shelf drugs
  caffeine content of, 25t
Onions
  triggering migraine, 24t
Opiates, 48, 56
Oppenheim, Hermann, 5
Orudis, 51t
Oruvail, 51t
Oxycodone, 48
OxyContin, 48

P
PA. *See* Physician assistant (PA)
Pain
  side-locked, 37
Pamate, 53t
Pamelor, 53t
Parentified children, 2
Paroxetine (Paxil), 53t
Patient doctor discussion, 11–12
Paxil, 53t
Peanut butter
  triggering migraine, 24t
Pepperoni
  triggering migraine, 24t
Petadolex, 44
Petasites hybridus (Butterbur), 44
Peters, Gustavus, 6
Phenelzine (Nardil), 53t
Physical examination, 10–11
Physical therapy, 46
  for neck pain, 36
Physician assistant (PA), 12
Pickled foods
  triggering migraine, 24t
Pizza
  triggering migraine, 24t
Ponstel, 51t
Post-concussion syndrome, 38
Post-traumatic headaches, 38
Posture, 27, 46f
  head and neck, 46
  head-forward, 27
Pregabalin (Lyrica), 41, 52t
Prescription medications
  caffeine content of, 25t
  preventive, 40–41
Preventive anti-epilepsy medications, 52t
Preventive medications
  headache calendars, 12
Preventive prescription medications, 40–41
Propranolol (Inderal), 40, 50t
Proton-pump inhibitors, 48
Protriptyline (Vivactil), 53t
Prozac, 40, 42, 50, 53t
Pseudotumor cerebri, 34

Q
Quality of life, 2

R
Rebound headaches, 6, 7
Red wine
  triggering migraine, 22, 24t
Relafen, 51t
Relpax, 48, 54t
Remeron, 53t
Riboflavin (vitamin B2), 44, 45
Rizatriptan (Maxalt), 48, 54t

S
Salami
  triggering migraine, 24t
Sausages
  triggering migraine, 24t
Scalp
  anatomy of, 19f
Scher, Anne, 27
Secondary headache, 29
Selective serotonin reuptake inhibitors (SSRI),
  42, 53t
  triggering migraine, 23t
Sensitive brain, 18
Serotonin, 19
  blockers, 42
Serotonin norepinephrine reuptake inhibitors, 53t
Serotonin syndrome, 50
Sertraline (Zoloft), 53t
Serzone, 53t
7-Up
  caffeine content of, 25t
Sexual activity, 2, 30
Side-locked pain, 37
Sinequan, 53t
Sinus disease, 34–36
Sinuses
  diagram of, 35f
Sinus headache, 35
Sinusitis
  acute, 35
  chronic, 36
  sphenoid, 35
Sleep, 2
Sneezing, 30
Snoring, 27t
Soft drinks
  caffeine content of, 25t
Sour cream
  triggering migraine, 24t
Specialists, 56
Sphenoid sinusitis, 35
Spinal manipulation
  for neck pain, 36
Spinal tap (lumbar puncture), 33
Splenda (sucralose)
  triggering migraine, 23t, 24t
SSRI. *See* Selective serotonin reuptake inhibitors
  (SSRI)
Stewart, Walter, 2
Stress, 26, 27t

Substance P, 43
Sucralose
  triggering migraine, 23t, 24t
Sugar substitute
  triggering migraine, 23t
Sullivan, Mary, 6
Sumatriptan (Imitrex), 48, 54t
Supplements, 44–45

T
Tanacetum parthenium, 44, 45
Tea
  caffeine content of, 25t
Telephones, 27
Temporomandibular joints (TMJ), 11, 27, 37, 47f
Tense jaw, 27
Tension-type headache, 5
  characteristics of, 9t
  classification of, 14
  connection with migraine, 28
  diagnosis of, 8–9
  triggers, 27
Tests, 10–11
Tetracycline
  triggering migraine, 23t
Thyroid disease, 27t
  causing headache, 27
Tiagabine (Gabitril), 52t
Timolol (Blocadren), 40, 50t
Tizanidine (Zanaflex), 40, 41
TMJ. *See* Temporomandibular joints (TMJ)
Tofranil, 53t
Topiramate (Topamax), 40, 41, 49, 50t, 52t
Toradol, 51t
Transformed migraine, 2
Tranylcypromine (Pamate), 53t
Trazodone (Desyrel), 53t
Trepanation, 4
Trephination, 4
Tricyclic antidepressants, 53t
Trigeminal (fifth cranial) nerve, 20
Trigeminovascular system
  anatomy of, 19f, 20
Trigger(s)
  caffeine, 26
  determining, 10, 12
  dietary, 24t
  elimination of, 47
  and Lyme disease, 27, 27t
  for migraines, 18, 22–23, 23t, 24f, 35

  neck and peripheral muscles, 21
  self-help techniques, 55
  tension-type headache, 27
Trigger points, 46
  injections, 22
  injections for neck pain, 36
Triptans, 54t
Tylenol, 23
Typing, 27
Tyramine
  triggering migraine, 23

U
Underlying medical conditions, 29–38

V
Vanquish
  caffeine content of, 25t
Venlafaxine (Effexor), 53t
Vicodin, 48
Viral infections, 27t, 30
Visual aura, 13
Vitamin(s), 44–45
Vitamin A
  triggering migraine, 23t
Vitamin B2, 44, 45
Vivactil, 53t
Vivarin tablets
  caffeine content of, 25t
Voltaren, 51t

W
Wellbutrin, 53t
Whiplash, 38
Willis, Thomas, 4–5
Worry, 29–38
Wörz, Roland, 6

Y
Yoga, 46
Yogurt
  triggering migraine, 24t

Z
Zanaflex, 40, 41
Zolmitriptan (Zomig), 48, 54t
Zoloft, 53t
Zomig, 48, 54t
Zonisamide (Zonegran), 52t